LIVING YOGA

A Comprehensive Guide for Daily Life

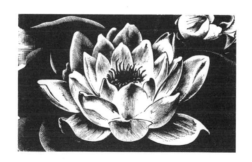

Edited by
GEORG FEUERSTEIN *and* STEPHAN BODIAN
with the staff of YOGA JOURNAL

A Jeremy P. Tarcher/Putnam Book
published by
G. P. PUTNAM'S SONS
New York

Most Tarcher/Putnam books are available at special quantity discounts for bulk purchases for sales promotions, premiums, fund-raising, and educational needs. Special books, or book excerpts, can also be created to fit specific needs.
For details, write or telephone Special Markets, Putnam Publishing Group, 200 Madison Avenue, New York, NY 10016. (212) 951-8891.

A Jeremy P. Tarcher/Putnam Book
Published by G. P. Putnam's Sons
Publishers Since 1838
200 Madison Avenue
New York, NY 10016

http://www.putnam.com/putnam

Published simultaneously in Canada

Library of Congress Cataloging-in-Publication Data

Living yoga: a comprehensive guide for daily life / edited by Georg Feuerstein and
    Stephan Bodian and the staff of *Yoga Journal*.
        p.   cm.
        Collection of articles originally published in *Yoga Journal*. Includes index.
        ISBN 0-87477-729-1 (pbk. : alk. paper)
        1. Yoga.   I. Feuerstein, Georg.   II. Bodian, Stephan.   III. *Yoga Journal*.
    B132.Y6L56   1993   92-35692 CIP
    181'.45—dc20

Design by Susan Shankin

Printed in the United States of America
        13 14 15 16 17 18 19 20

For copyrights and permissions, see page 277.

This book is printed on acid-free paper.

Contents

PART ONE
Cultivating the Body: Hatha Yoga

PART TWO
Transcending the Mind: Raja Yoga

Acknowledgments

We would like to thank all the writers who have contributed to *Yoga Journal* over the years, especially those whose work appears in these pages. Without their generous and enthusiastic involvement, neither this book nor the magazine would ever have been possible.

Our thanks also to the loyal readers of our magazine, who share our love of yoga and have sustained and inspired us for nearly two decades.

Finally, we would like to express our deepest appreciations to the staff of *Yoga Journal* for keeping the vision alive, and especially to our publisher, Michael Gliksohn, whose integrity and dedication have carried us forward over the years; our former managing editor, Linda Cogozzo; our art director, Larry Watson; our associate editor, Anne Cushman; and our assistant editor, Holly Hammond, who worked long hours amassing the photos and organizing the materials for this book. Their devotion to the values that yoga exemplifies is reflected in every page.

Preface

In the popular imagination, yoga and meditation are still associated with the counterculture of the 1960s. In fact, however, America's fascination with the wisdom of the East has a long and illustrious history. As early as the 1840s, American transcendentalists, such as Emerson and Thoreau, were reading and discussing the *Bhagavad Gita*, one of yoga's core sacred texts. Thoreau even wrote about practicing yoga (no doubt of an intellectual variety) and at one point characterized himself as "to some extent . . . a yogi."

In the 1870s the Theosophical Society, which preached a blend of Hinduism, Buddhism, and Western esotericism, was founded in New York City. By the 1890s it had over fifty U.S. branches.

But it was not until 1893, when Swami Vivekananda, a disciple of the renowned Indian sage Ramakrishna, gave a much-heralded talk at the World Parliament of Religions in Chicago that yoga as a practice actually began to take root on this continent. Although Vivekananda didn't teach the postures for which yoga has become famous, he did have eager Western adepts of a century ago sitting cross-legged and focusing their attention in meditation. By the time Vivekananda died in 1902, the Vedanta centers he had founded in several U.S. cities were well established, and the young yoga sapling had already started to flourish in American soil.

Today we are harvesting the fruit of this 100-year efflorescence. Inspired and enriched by a steady influx of Eastern teachers, yoga has penetrated the mainstream during the past several decades. Throughout the U.S., health clubs, fitness salons, and community centers offer hatha yoga classes as a much sought-after adjunct to aerobic exercise, weight training, and a fast-paced life-style in general. Stress-reduction and healing techniques based on the teachings of yoga have attracted the attention of physicians and therapists and are now standard practice at many hospitals and clinics. And the philosophy of yoga and the related traditions of Buddhism and Taoism have had an immeasurable impact on contemporary Western art, music, literature, environmentalism, and psychology. Even media giants like *Newsweek* and the *Washington Post*, which are often slow to acknowledge the influence of alternative trends, have recently touted the benefits of yoga.

Since 1975, *Yoga Journal* has covered American yoga in all its breadth, from dietary regimes to transpersonal psychology, from stress-reduction techniques to deep ecology, from therapeutic yoga to the teachings of contemporary sages. Many of the articles that have appeared on our pages have provided information and inspiration of timeless value. Over the years we've watched with more than a little regret as each issue has come and gone, carrying with it into a kind of journalistic limbo the valuable wisdom it contains.

Now, with the encouragement of Jeremy Tarcher and his staff, we've gathered some of this material into a single volume, woven together by the insightful essays of co-editor Georg Feuerstein. While not pretending to be an exhaustive overview of contemporary yoga, this book provides the interested reader with a sampling of the many yoga and yoga-inspired teachings and practices now available in the West.

Organized according to the six primary branches of yoga—hatha, raja, bhakti, karma, tantra, and jnana—the book is designed to appeal to neophytes and to those who are already practicing yoga. Beginners will find it to be a wide-ranging yet accessible reader, with listings of books and organizations for those who wish to pursue further study. Seasoned practitioners will be pleased to discover a wealth of original material by luminaries in the fields of yoga, health, and spirituality, including *Yoga Journal* regulars Donald Moyer, Judith Lasater, Mary Schatz, and Donna Farhi, as well as prominent teachers and healers such as Ram Dass, Joan Borysenko, Joanna Macy, and Ken Wilber. And, of course, fans of the magazine will now have access to a compendium of the best articles published during the past decade.

As editor of *Yoga Journal* since 1984, I've had the pleasure of working closely with all of the writers whose work appears here. As the volume took shape under Georg Feuerstein's able direction, I found myself reading over articles I hadn't seen in years and marveling at their quality.

"What a fine magazine we've been publishing!" I mused, with perhaps a bit more than my fair share of pride. I'm thrilled to see this valuable material find a more permanent home at last. And I hope that in its store of information you will find a few pearls of wisdom to guide and inspire you on your own personal journey.

Stephan Bodian
Berkeley, California
September 1992

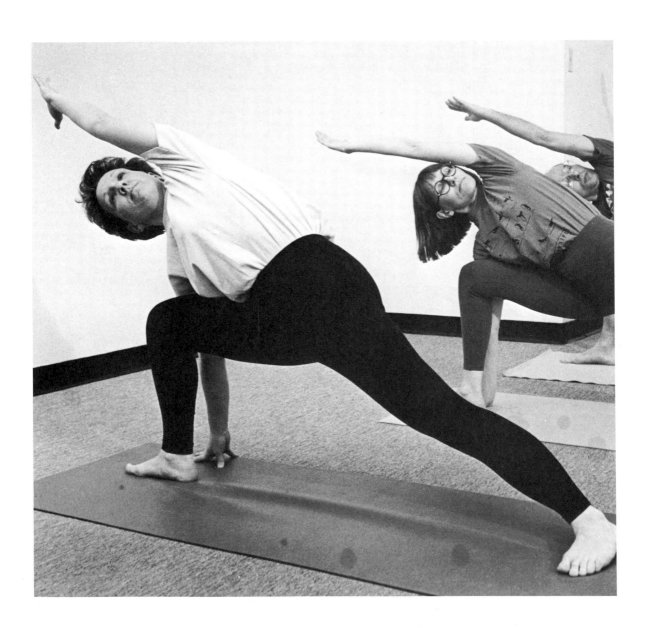

ONE

Introducing Yoga
by Georg Feuerstein, Ph.D.

YOGA IN THE WEST

Yoga has become a household word in the West. Millions of men and women have read books about yoga, attended classes or seminars, and experimented with the physical exercises for which yoga is famous. Millions more have tried meditation, and many continue to practice some form of yoga on a regular basis.

Clearly, the yogic tradition is far from being a fossilized relic from a remote past and distant country. Yoga is very much alive in Western society, and its prospects for further growth are excellent.

In fact, by now yoga has its own distinct heritage in Europe and America—a heritage that is exactly 100 years old in 1993. For it was in 1893 that one of India's celebrated sages, Swami Vivekananda, was applauded by thousands at the World Fair in Chicago. More than anyone, this charismatic figure stimulated the West's interest in yoga and opened the gates to a never-ending stream of yogis and swamis from India.

Ah, we live joyously, without hate among those who hate! Among people who hate we dwell without hate.

Ah, we live joyously, in health among those who are afflicted! Among people who are afflicted, we dwell in health.

Ah, we live joyously, in peace, among those who struggle! Among people who struggle we live in peace.

DHAMMAPADA, 197–199

WHAT DOES "YOGA" MEAN?

The word *yoga* stems from the Sanskrit language, in which the sacred scriptures of Hinduism are composed. It means "union" but also "discipline." Combining these two connotations, we can define yoga as "unitive discipline"—the discipline that leads to inner and outer union, harmony, and joy.

Whether we know it or not, we all seek to maximize our well-being and joy. However, sometimes we try to do so in strange and self-destructive ways, mainly because we confuse pleasure and immediate satisfaction with abiding happiness and fulfillment. Thus, people turn to quick fixes like alcohol, drugs, and sex. They run the risk of becoming addicts and undermining their health, relationships, and livelihood. Addicts are essentially people who have failed to learn the principal lesson of yoga: Happiness cannot be bought with a quick fix but is the mature fruit of a life dedicated to higher values and ideals.

Yoga is first and foremost the discipline of conscious living. When we take charge of our lives, we also tap into our inner potential for happiness, or what in Sanskrit is called *ananda*. This primal joy, which transcends the ego or personality, wells up in our hearts and infuses our whole being with vibrant energy—*life*. Thus energized, or enlivened, we can go about the business of our daily living in a harmonious manner. We become highly creative, establishing order where there is chaos; instilling life where there is a vacuum; causing comfort where there is distress. In other words, because we are full of joy and life, we become a healing presence in the world.

Our external reality is a reflection of our inner reality. When we are unhappy and depressed, not only does everything look bleak to us, but we also subtly affect our environment. When people around us sense our gloominess, they tend to react in less than happy ways. They may get angry, or take on our depression, or simply avoid us. Unhappiness is contagious; it rubs off on others.

But so does happiness. For instance, when you are in love and the world looks radiant, beautiful, and perfect, you want to embrace every stranger and draw him or her into your magic circle of happiness. You smile at people and, with few exceptions, they smile back at you. Like a high-voltage spark, your happiness arcs across to them, igniting their own inner joy.

In the famous Arabic story of Laila and Majnun—the Middle Eastern equivalent of Romeo and Juliet—Majnun is given ample opportunity to fall in love with many girls more beautiful than Laila. But he only loves Laila and thinks her the most beautiful of all. He imbues her with beauty or, rather, he sees beyond her human form to her inner beauty. In other words, his love reaches out to seek the love within her, to touch her in the depth of her own joy.

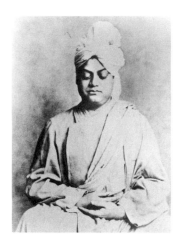

SWAMI VIVEKANANDA

Majnun explains that the form does not matter, only the essence. He compares Laila to the wine in a cup. He is indifferent to the cup but partial to its content. Even a gem-studded chalice would be useless if it contained vinegar instead of wine.

In his perception of the world, Majnun penetrates deep beneath the surface. This is the task and virtue of all sages: They look deeper than the ordinary person. Yoga seeks to promote that depth perception or communion with reality. The yogis learn to look upon the world with new eyes—the eyes of joy, love, and harmony. They not only see things differently from the ordinary individual; they *are* different. They live in an extraordinary state of being, which has been given such labels as "liberation," "freedom," "perfect spontaneity," and "Self-realization."

Unfortunately, in our civilization we are not taught to cultivate love and happiness and the singular state of being from which they spring. Rather, everything around us conspires to hide that possibility from us. In our schools, colleges, and universities we are not taught how we might get in touch with our innermost potential. For the most part, teachers are as unhappy as their students. There is a widespread ban on happiness and ecstasy.

Nevertheless, we recognize happiness when we encounter it. It is not an alien experience for us, merely a rare one. Bobby McFerrin's little tune "Don't Worry, Be Happy"—a phrase borrowed from Meher Baba, one of modern India's great miracle-working saints—was an instant success when it was aired on the radio. Its simple lyrics and melody captured something of the spirit of happiness, which is suppressed in us most of the time.

Like McFerrin's tune, yoga practice is a means of contacting our inner happiness. But there is an important difference: When we are cheered up by listening to a song or by receiving a happy message, we are entirely passive. However, in yoga practice we put spectatorship to rest and actively promote our own happiness and well-being. We take charge of our own cure for unhappiness. We are the remedy.

In laughter, we transcend our predicaments.

ALLEN KLEIN

A distinction should be made between yogism and Yoga, between an ensemble of techniques whose purpose is to give a man balance, to relax him and to free him from various complexes, and that whole which is Yoga, which seeks to make the body the instrument of the interior man, and the interior man an enlightened guide for the body.

J. M. DECHANET

YOGA: WHAT IT IS AND WHAT IT IS NOT

Some people think that yoga is calisthenics, epitomized by the headstand, the lotus posture, or another pretzel-like pose. Others think it is a system of meditation. Yet others regard it, perhaps fearfully, as a religion. All these stereotypes are misleading. It is true that some branches of yoga—notably hatha yoga—involve numerous postures (asana).

However, these are not merely somatic exercises but are meant to be practiced in the larger context of a life of conscious spiritual discipline. Also, at the core of almost all schools of yoga lies the practice of meditation. However, yoga is much more than meditation; it is a way of life. While it contains ideas, prescriptions, and practices that can be found in religious traditions, yoga entails a practical, experimental approach that is not based on belief. Its pragmatism is quite unique.

Yoga seeks to give us a new sense of identity by enlarging our inner horizon. Alan Watts put it well when he observed: "We do not need a new religion or a new bible. We need a new experience—a new feeling of what it is to be 'I'."[1] Through the disciplines of yoga, we can acquire a new self-perception or self-understanding. We can find out who we really are.

Our civilization has a strong taboo against such self-knowledge. We are encouraged to learn any number of facts about the world—a process we call education. But we are not encouraged to turn the same inquisitiveness toward ourselves. Even classes in psychology, by and large, are about external aspects of the human mind. So, many young people who choose to study psychology in order to discover themselves are disappointed and may abandon their courses.

Anyone who is bold or desperate enough to challenge that taboo, venturing forth into the treacherous waters of self-discovery, invites ridicule and possibly ostracism. It is considered insane not to accept the standard definition of who we are. And what is that? We are, so the myth goes, the "normal," insular ego-personality that goes about its daily business of eating, drinking, sleeping, working and having sex—which Watts labeled the "meat tube."

But this view of human nature is appallingly inadequate and untrue. A vastly different image of human nature has for millennia been entertained in the great spiritual traditions of the world. These traditions are grounded not merely on hopeful ideas and well-meaning ideals but on a range of significant experiences that are almost completely denied by scientific materialism. These experiences include lucid dreaming, out-of-body states, clairvoyance, and other psychic abilities, as well as ecstasies, mystical states and, at the apex of them all, enlightenment.

Yoga is at home with all these mental states and mind-transcending realizations. All genuine yoga is concerned with enlightenment, which is spoken of in different terms: Self-realization, God-realization, mystical union, communion with Reality, ultimate self-transcendence, awakening to the higher Being, the condition of unconditional love, the attainment of perfect peace, the realization of unalloyed bliss, and so on.

In addition to this supreme value or ideal, yoga also recognizes a variety of secondary goals, such as physical well-being, moral integrity, and social service and harmony. Some forms of yoga seem at first glance to be more concerned with one or the other secondary goal. For instance, hatha yoga is widely taught as the cultivation of bodily health, including vigor and suppleness. Raja yoga is commonly presented as an approach for cultivating the mind's potential for concentration and meditation. However, both hatha yoga and raja yoga, as well as other authentic schools of yoga, operate within a larger framework that recognizes Self-realization, or enlightenment, as the principal ideal.

Growing is the most important and essential endeavor that a human being can undertake.

SWAMI CHETANANANDA

According to the yoga tradition, enlightenment is the summit of the vast mountain we call human existence. Most people are content with traveling in the valley, barely aware of the awesome peak and its possibilities, which extend into the sky. Some people like to hike up its slopes occasionally, breathing the cleaner, cooler air. Or they may glance up at the summit now and then but are intimidated by its distance.

Then there are those few who are serious about climbing the slopes and scaling the outcrops, going beyond the treeline and across the ice pack. They are spurred on in their efforts by the great ones on the summit the illumined sages who live in perpetual bliss and peace. From their vantage point, they calmly but compassionately behold the busy people in the valley, blessing everyone and patiently waiting for those who follow their footsteps up the mountain.

Sometimes a few of them take it upon themselves to come down from their quiet retreat in the bright light of the eternal sun in order to mix with the folk in the noisy marketplace. They bring the summit's peace and tranquility with them, and now and then they succeed in awakening others and attracting them to explore the hidden glories of the mountain.

YOGA IS A UNIVERSAL ART

The great teachers, or gurus, were the ingenious inventors of the yoga tradition with its incredible store of methods, techniques, moral attitudes, and ideas. Although yoga originated within the fold of Hinduism, it cannot be equated with that religion. It is more an art—the art of living at the highest level possible for a human being, in attunement with the larger life—Reality with a capital R.

Admittedly, many aspects of yoga have a Hindu flavor, such as the Sanskrit mantras (sacred sounds) that practitioners may recite aloud or repeat mentally, or the ideas of moral retribution (karma) and reincarnation. However, the emphasis in yoga is always on experimentation and personal verification rather than mere belief. Besides, some of the ideas that may seem typically Hindu and possibly strike you as strange, such as reincarnation, are not unique to Hinduism. The premise that life continues after the death of the physical body and that our spiritual identity is subsequently clothed in another body is common to many religious traditions.

Of course, most Hindus take this as a matter of unquestioned dogma. But we can easily practice yoga without it. It is interesting to note, however, that many intelligent Westerners who have considered the possibility of reincarnation have been struck by its explanatory value. Among them are such illustrious personages as Pythagoras, Plato, Plotinus, Nietzsche, Emerson, and Yeats.

Yoga is indeed associated with certain metaphysical notions, but the practice itself does not require that we adopt them. People of any religious or spiritual persuasion, as well as open-minded agnostics, can practice yoga with great benefit. Ultimately, however, they tend to have the kinds of yogic experiences that cause them at least to entertain, if not adopt, the theories offered by the yoga tradition. And these theories are diverse, allowing plenty of room for intellectual creativity and questioning.

If this sounds strange to some ears, we merely need to point out the case of Gautama the Buddha, who lived some 2,500 years ago. Although brought up in the Hindu tradition, he was really an agnostic of sorts. He refused to speculate about ultimate things and advised his disciples to simply tread the path he had discovered and walked before them.

So, the metaphysical explanations of yoga should not prove a stumbling block to anyone with a genuine desire to explore this ancient tradition. It is this built-in flexibility that has allowed the yoga tradition to adapt itself so well to the conditions of the West. It can be as meaningful for nondogmatic agnostics, Christians, or Jews as it is for Hindus.

Yoga, then, is a universal art, which flourishes wherever a person is dedicated to higher values, to a way of life that outdistances the egotistical preoccupations of the unenlightened mind: the way of inner joy and outer harmony.

Treading a Way does not consist in mechanically applying a technique until liberation is achieved. There are no magic formulas or assembly-line techniques. Each person must come up with his or her own Way—by giving up most dearly held convictions and habits, by making use of all resources, by doing the most extraordinary spiritual somersault.

PIERO FERRUCCI

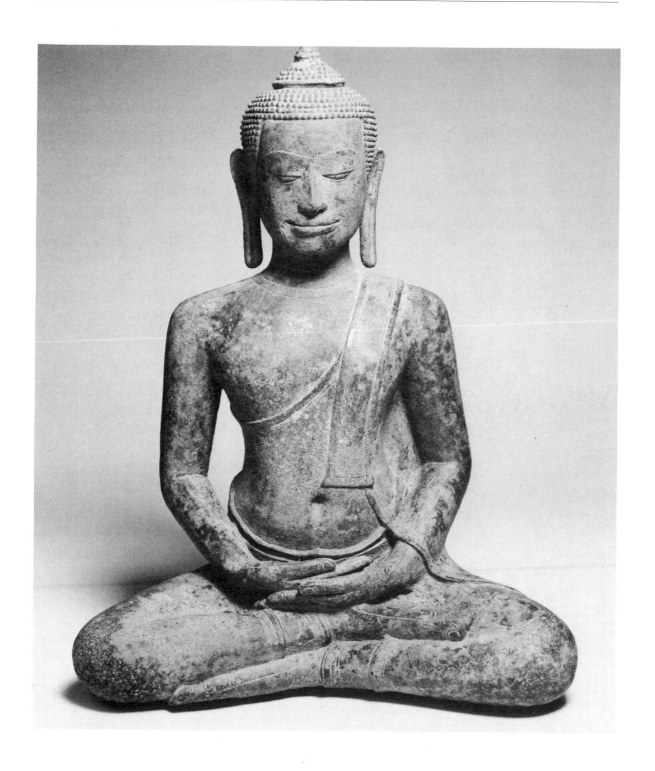

THE MAJOR BRANCHES OF THE TREE OF YOGA

You can picture yoga as a tree that is 5,000 and more years old. It has big tangled roots, a gigantic stem, several huge branches, numerous secondary branches, and countless twigs. Some of the branches are quite dead, while others are very much alive, blossoming anew every spring.

There are six major branches of yoga: hatha yoga, raja yoga, karma yoga, bhakti yoga, jnana yoga, and tantra yoga. Each branch is suited for a different personality style or approach to life. Hatha yoga is the "forceful" (hatha) path, involving the deliberate arousal of the body's psychospiritual energy, called *kundalini shakti* or "serpent power." It is this energy that is thought to rise through the seven primary psychospiritual centers (chakras or cakras) of the body. Its journey ends at the crown center at the top of the head and coincides with the experience of ecstasy without a trace of duality in consciousness.

Traditionally, this path called for tremendous courage, determination, and physical fitness. The modern Western approach to hatha yoga is less demanding, and in fact is widely employed as a form of physical therapy.

Raja yoga is the "royal" (raja) path, proceeding by means of meditation and inner and outer renunciation. This approach is identical with classical yoga, as outlined in the *Yoga Sutra* of Patanjali, composed sometime in the first or second century A.D., or, according to some authorities, even earlier. Raja yoga consists of the well-known eight "limbs": moral discipline, self-restraint, posture, breath control, sensory inhibition, concentration, meditation, and ecstasy. These components are found in many other branches of yoga as well.

Raja yoga calls for an ability to turn inward and exercise a high degree of discernment and dispassion. Individuals who can concentrate well and enjoy meditation are best suited for this yogic approach.

Karma yoga is the path of self-transcending action, as taught in the *Bhagavad Gita*, the New Testament of Hinduism. So long as we act out of egotism, without awareness of our true spiritual identity, action (karma) is thought to bind consciousness. In other words, such action is "karmic." It leads to desire, which leads to other actions of a similar nature, which obscure our true identity more and more. Karma yoga seeks to break this vicious cycle and guide us to spiritual freedom through the discipline of work that is selfless and performed as a service to others.

This is the aim of Yoga: the elevation of the narrow, fear-ridden and desire-tormented human consciousness to a state of indescribable beauty, glory, and bliss.

GOPI KRISHNA

Since fierce asceticism, practiced in remote caves and forests, is not part of the modern Western way of life, karma yoga can be said to apply to virtually all yoga practitioners in the contemporary world. It can bring sanity and balance to our work-oriented society.

Bhakti yoga is the path of self-transcending devotion or all-embracing love for the Divine, which is seen as being present in every person and thing. This is often considered to be the easiest approach. However, for it to bear spiritual fruit, our devotion or love must be intense and pure. Bhakti yoga is best suited for those who are emotionally fluid and seek to cultivate an open heart.

Jnana yoga is the path of discernment and wisdom, as taught in the *Upanishads*. The crucial exercise of discernment, which distinguishes the Real from the unreal, or true happiness from fleeting pleasure, is supported by inner and outer renunciation. This is the path of the sage, who has understood that the spiritual process is a matter of simply dispelling the illusion that we are no more than the limited body-mind. The sage's approach is the most direct but also the most difficult, calling for a high degree of wisdom and inner detachment.

Jnana yoga calls for more than intellectual acumen, and it is not for beginners. However, those gifted with a mind capable of higher intuition and discernment can include jnana yoga in their spiritual life.

Tantra yoga is the path of self-transcendence through ritual means, including consecrated sexuality. The fundamental axiom of tantra yoga, or Tantrism, is that there is no real gap between the Divine and the world, but that the Divine inheres in the world and, therefore, can be found in the midst of ordinary life. Today tantra yoga is widely misunderstood as consisting exclusively of sexual rituals, and many Westerners are attracted to this branch of yoga because of that assumption. However, genuine tantra yoga involves a great deal more than sex, and in fact most tantric schools recommend a celibate life-style.

Tantra yoga is the most "Oriental" and esoteric of all yogic branches. However, some of its ideas and rituals may be found meaningful by Western yoga practitioners. It is best suited for those serious students of yoga who have an inner relationship to the feminine cosmic principle (Shakti) and who enjoy a more ceremonial approach.

Yoga Today

Life in Western society is more complex than at any other time in history. It is certainly far more complex than the traditional society of

It is impossible to disregard one of India's greatest discoveries: that of consciousness as witness, of consciousness freed from its psychological structures and their temporal conditioning, the consciousness of the "liberated" man.

Mircea Eliade

Much of Oriental philosophy is more sane than anything the West has produced.

Gregory Bateson

9

India, yoga's homeland. This fact clearly needs to be taken into account when we practice yoga in the West.

Since 1975, the editors of *Yoga Journal* have endeavored to find ways of communicating genuine yogic teachings in the context of modern life. While Westerners and Easterners have much in common in regard to their aptitude for the yogic path, there are certain significant differences that need to be addressed.

On the simplest level, we in the West are brought up to sit on chairs, whereas the Indians are accustomed to sitting cross-legged, which makes it easier for them to learn some of the yogic postures.

We are accustomed to questioning authority (though perhaps not enough and not with the necessary respect), but in India people are taught early on to accept authority—whether secular or religious—almost blindly. This can lead to slavish imitation of teachers and blind faith but also, occasionally, to exemplary devotedness to the guru. In the West, discipleship presents something of a problem for most people. We tend to cultivate doubt rather than trust, and this can be a big stumbling block on the spiritual path. While we can dispense with mere belief, trust is essential to a wholesome life.

Our dietary habits are by and large detrimental to our well-being. Most Indians are vegetarians and, because they do not enjoy the same affluence, they also eat more moderately. Their adoption of a yogic way of life is thus far less dramatic and traumatic. In the West, however, anyone who seriously wants to practice yoga must summon a great deal of energy to reverse ingrained dietary and other life-style habits.

Finally, to mention one other important difference, yoga is an integral part of the Hindu culture. The whole outlook of yoga is not alien for Indians, as it tends to be for Westerners who, after all, are directly or indirectly conditioned by the attitudes and values of Christianity and Judaism.

These differences are not necessarily disadvantageous for Western students of yoga. In some cases, they can even be of considerable advantage. However, they demand a reinterpretation of yoga for contemporary Westerners. *Yoga Journal* has endeavored to do just that by bringing the yoga tradition into contact with modern Western developments in psychology, medicine, and healthcare.

This book, which is largely a compendium of articles that originally appeared in *Yoga Journal*, adopts the same approach. In these pages, you will find articles and interviews that do not directly relate to the yoga tradition as we have defined it here. Rather, the guiding principle

It is the great tragedy of contemporary Western society that we have virtually lost the ability to experience the transformative power of ecstasy and joy.

ROBERT A. JOHNSON

Even adults have numerous possibilities for change.

DON JOHNSON

of the magazine's editor (co-editor of this book), Stephan Bodian, has been to include articles that reflect, more broadly, "the qualities of being that yoga exemplifies: peace, integrity, clarity, and compassion." This material will, we believe, provide a helpful context for your personal practice of yoga.

RESOURCES

Books

Eliade, M. *Patanjali and Yoga.* New York: Schocken Books, 1975. This is an introductory work, based on the author's comprehensive study (see following note).

_____. *Yoga: Immortality and Freedom.* Princeton, NJ: Princeton University Press, 1973. A classic scholarly treatment of yoga and associated traditions.

Feuerstein, G. *Encyclopedic Dictionary of Yoga.* New York: Paragon House, 1990. The most comprehensive illustrated encyclopedia on yoga, covering all its aspects.

_____. *Yoga: The Technology of Ecstasy.* Los Angeles: J. P. Tarcher, 1986. The most comprehensive overview of the yoga tradition available today. It covers the history, philosophy, literature, and practice of yoga.

Iyengar, B. K. S. *The Tree of Yoga.* Boston, MA: Shambhala, 1989. This is an informative and wise introduction to yoga practice by an accomplished yogi and world-renowned teacher of hatha yoga.

Manos, M., ed. *Iyengar: His Life and Work.* Porthill, ID: Timeless Books, 1987. This anthology is a tribute to Sri B. K. S. Iyengar.

Sri Chinmoy. *Yoga and the Spiritual Life: The Journey of India's Soul.* Jamaica, NY: Agni Press, 1974. A lively introduction to yogic spirituality by a renowned adept.

Swami Chetananda. *The Breath of God.* Cambridge, MA: Rudra Press, 1973. A practical introduction to the spiritual side of yoga, written by a respected teacher.

Periodicals

Journal of the International Association of Yoga Therapists is published twice a year. Subscription address: IAYT, 4150 Tivoli Avenue, Los Angeles, CA 90066.

Light of Consciousness: Chit Jyoti, a quarterly publication, is published by Truth Consciousness, founded by Swami Amar Jyoti. It is dedicated to the theme of spiritual awakening and Self-realization. Subscription and editorial address: 10668 Gold Hill Road, Boulder, CO 80302-9716.

Quest, a quarterly magazine, is published by the Theosophical Society in America. It often features articles of relevance to yoga practitioners. Subscription and editorial address: P.O. Box 270, Wheaton, IL 60189.

Yoga International, a young publication, is published six times a year by the Himalayan International Institute in conjunction with Yoga International, Inc. Subscription and editorial address: Himalayan Institute, RDI, Box 88 Honesdale, PA 18431.

Yoga Journal is a bimonthly publication established by the California Yoga Teachers Association, a nonprofit California educational corporation. This is the most widely read magazine on yoga. Subscription address: P.O. Box 469018, Escondido, CA 92046. Editorial address: 2054 University Avenue, Berkeley, CA 94704.

Organizations

Unity in Yoga is an organization, headed by Nancy Ford-Kohne, which is dedicated to promoting unity among the various schools of yoga. This organization, which is deliberately eclectic in its orientation, sponsors large biannual conferences. Unity in Yoga can be contacted at: 7918 Bolling Drive, Alexandria, VA 22308. Tel. (703) 765-7707.

International Association of Yoga Therapists, founded in 1989, sponsors medical and psychological research on yoga and publishes a semiannual journal featuring technical articles. Membership includes subscription to the journal. Address: IAYT, 4150 Tivoli Avenue, Los Angeles, CA 90066.

Spiritual Emergence Network (SEN), founded in 1980 by Christina Grof, is an international organization that seeks to help individuals undergoing spiritual emergencies, such as kundalini awakenings and nonordinary states of consciousness. This organization has over 1000 volunteers—both professionals and lay people—and handles an average of 150 callers a month. The address is: 5905 Soquel #650, Soquel, CA 95073. Tel. (510) 464-8261.

Note

[1] A. Watts, *The Book: On the Taboo Against Knowing Who You Are* (New York: Vintage Books, 1972), p. 11.

PART ONE

CULTIVATING THE BODY: HATHA YOGA

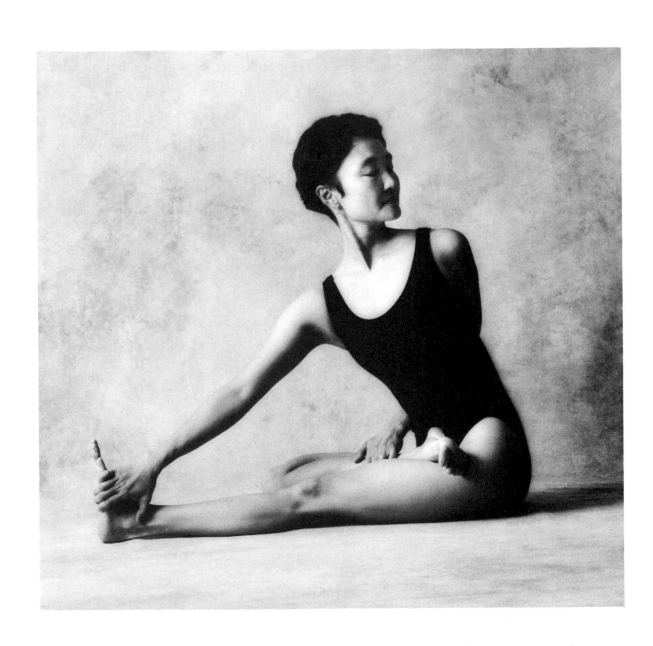

TWO

Getting Started with Yoga

The first chapter served as an introduction to the overall purpose and outlook of the yoga tradition. In this chapter you will learn about some of the fundamental principles of yoga practice.

The contributions here contain concrete guidelines that will enable you to practice yoga wisely and successfully. This includes a gentle but firm approach to discipline and how to enlist the aid of the body's most powerful mechanism for personal change: the breath, which is an aspect of the universal life-force (prana). The chapter begins with a brief consideration of the place of hatha yoga in the yogic tradition as a whole.

Of what is the body made? It is made of emptiness and rhythm. At the ultimate heart of the body, at the heart of the world, there is no solidity. Once again, there is only the dance.

GEORGE LEONARD

HATHA YOGA AND THE EIGHTFOLD PATH

Hatha yoga represents a particular phase in the evolution of the yoga tradition and is based on the eightfold path outlined by Patanjali in his *Yoga Sutra*. Hatha yoga dates back to the eleventh century A.D., when Gorakshanatha, a great master, articulated its philosophy and also discovered many of the hatha yoga practices. It is the distilled experience of more than four millennia of yogic experimentation.

The teachers of hatha yoga recognize the eight steps of Patanjali's path, but have greatly elaborated two of them—posture and breath control. In its classical form, the path of yoga is made up of the following eight steps: moral observances (including virtues such as nonharming, truthfulness, nonstealing, chastity, and greedlessness), self-discipline

15

Hatha Yoga is a method that will achieve the maximum results by the minimum expenditure of energy.

THEOS BERNARD

(including purity, contentment, austerity, self-study, and devotion to a higher spiritual reality), posture, breath control, sensory inhibition, concentration, meditation, and ecstasy.

These eight steps lead to progressively deeper levels of awareness and functioning until, finally, ordinary consciousness is transcended in the bliss of ecstasy. In this elevated condition, we become one with the object of our contemplation, whether it be a physical form or the formless reality behind all forms. At the highest level of ecstasy, our true nature shines forth, and we realize that we are intrinsically free beings. This realization of freedom and joy is the great goal of all yogic traditions and schools, including hatha yoga, which is the one best known in the West.

Hatha yoga was invented to serve the spiritual needs of people living in what the Hindus call the *kali-yuga*, the Dark Age of spiritual decline, which is still in effect today. The adepts of hatha yoga felt that most people are too distracted to devote themselves wholeheartedly and effectively to the spiritual process, and that they require concrete aids to prepare the body-mind for the higher practices of meditation and ecstatic self-transcendence. So, they elaborated the third and fourth limb of the eightfold path taught by Patanjali, namely posture (asana) and breath control (pranayama).

Hatha yoga, as the Sanskrit name suggests, is the "powerful" path of realization. It seeks to awaken the body's inherent psychospiritual energy (called *kundalini*), which is thought to strengthen, heal, rejuvenate, and supercharge our physical frame. The reasoning behind this approach is that the advanced practices of yoga, such as meditation and ecstasy, require a strong and healthy body. *Mens sana in corpore sano,* "a sound mind in a sound body," as the Latin writer Juvenal put it.

Adepts of hatha yoga have demonstrated incredible control over their bodies. As laboratory tests bear out, they can stop their hearts, enter into a state of suspended animation, and regulate their brain waves at will. But astonishing as these feats are, they are not important in themselves. Rather they suggest that the great masters of yoga have access to a level of consciousness that is closed to most other people. They are in touch with the hidden dimension of existence, which, they assure us, is far richer, more joyous, and more rewarding than the experiences of ordinary life.

They also tell us that everyone can gain access to that same level of reality, providing they diligently apply themselves to the practice of yoga. Clearly, the yogic path is a lifelong endeavor, but this should encourage rather than discourage us. For we do not need to be in a big hurry. As the scriptures of yoga affirm, no effort is lost on the path. However, we must be willing to take the first step, then the next, and the next.

RESOURCES

Books

Feuerstein, G. *The Yoga-Sutra of Patanjali: A New Translation and Commentary*. Rochester, VT: Inner Traditions, 1989. This translation includes a word-by-word explanation of Patanjali's 195 aphorisms.

Ghosh, S. *The Original Yoga*. New Delhi: Munshiram Manoharlal, 1979. This work contains English translations of two important texts on hatha yoga—the *Gheranda Samhita* and the *Shiva Samhita*—as well as a rendering of the *Yoga Sutra*.

Iyengar, B. K. S. *Light on Yoga*. New York: Schocken Books, 1966. A yoga classic, with numerous illustrations.

Rieker, H.–U *The Yoga of Light*. Clearlake, CA: Dawn Horse Press, 1974. An annotated translation of the *Hatha Yoga Pradipika*, which is the most widely used Sanskrit text on hatha yoga.

Swami Sivananda Radha. *Hatha Yoga: The Hidden Language*. Foreword by B. K. S. Iyengar. Porthill, ID: Timeless Books, 1987. A sensitive study of the symbolic dimension of some hatha yoga postures.

Organizations

To find out about yoga classes in your area, you may consult the annual directory of yoga teachers published by *Yoga Journal*. The directory can be found in the July/August issue every year.

For yoga props, such as mats, outfits, etc., you may refer to the advertising section in *Yoga Journal*.

Yoga Journal also provides a book and tape service for readers. Another good source for yoga books, including some hard-to-find titles, is Open Secret, 923 C Street, San Rafael, CA 94901. Tel. (415) 457-4191.

Six Illusions About the Body
by Larry Dossey, M.D.

Most of us suffer from six illusions about the body. These misconceptions profoundly affect the way we relate to our body and to other beings.

1. *The body is solid.* In reality, most of the body is sheer vacuum.

2. *The body is stable.* In reality, our body is constantly changing. Every five years, all the cells have been replaced.

3. *The body is individuated.* In reality, we are in constant molecular exchange with other bodies, which makes nonsense out of the common presumption that a particular body is ours.

4. *The body belongs to the Earth.* In reality, the human body is made not simply of the maternal ovum and the paternal sperm, but of the high-energy material present at the Big Bang fourteen billion years ago.

5. *The body is stationary.* In reality, our body is never still but continuously in motion, together with all the other bodies, small or large, in the universe.

6. *The body is mindless.* In reality, far from being unconscious, our body is endowed with sentience apart from the functions of the brain. In other words, the brain is not the only "mindful" organ of the body. Tissues and organs far removed from the brain seem to have brainlike properties as well.

Resources

Books

Brunton, P. *The Body.* Burdett, NY: Larson Publications, 1986.

Dossey, L. *Meaning and Medicine.* New York: Bantam Books, 1991.

Murphy, M. *The Future of the Body: Explorations into the Further Evolution of Human Nature.* Los Angeles: J. P. Tarcher, 1992. A breathtaking survey of research and literature on the extraordinary capacities of the body—from stigmata to levitation.

COMING TO TERMS WITH EMBODIMENT

To be born means to be embodied. At the moment of death, our embodiment in the physical realm terminates. But from the moment of our first breath to the moment of our last, we live *in* and *as* our body. So, we must come to terms with our embodiment, with ourselves. If we fail to do so, we reduce our aliveness, cutting off the life force within us. That is, we choose death over life. So long as we are in conflict with our body, we cannot find peace of mind.

The human body is a wondrous thing.

RALPH STRAUCH

When we accept our embodiment, we also can embrace the world. When body and world cease to be enemies, there is joy. That joy is felt as vibrant life. In that joy, we expand beyond our apparent physical boundaries and get a sense that all of existence is just a single Body.

Being embodied is a unique opportunity to transmute matter into energy: to bring down the higher light, the radiance of the Self, into our seemingly dense physical vehicles. As the Indian philosopher-sage Sri Aurobindo put it: "As the crust of the outer nature cracks, as the walls of inner separation break down, the inner light gets through, the inner fire burns in the heart, the substance of the nature and the stuff of consciousness refine to a greater subtlety and purity . . . all is purified, set right, the whole nature harmonised, modulated in the psychic key, put in spiritual order."[1]

Thus we can become true alchemists, transforming a small but significant segment of the cosmos—our individual body-mind. This transformation will send benign ripples throughout the universe, for we know today, through the findings of physics, that everything is interconnected and that, therefore, even our least thoughts and actions affect the whole fabric of existence.

Our embodiment is thus not only a rare opportunity but also a great responsibility.

DEVELOPING YOUR OWN YOGA PRACTICE
BY HART LAZER

Why Practice?

We expend energy in many ways. We talk with our friends and loved ones, go to work, hurry from place to place and from task to task, with little time left to feel and respond to our bodies and our beings as a whole. Consequently, we often operate out of reflex conditioning or feelings of duty and responsibility.

This overloading tends to manifest itself as resentments and frustrations that lead us to act in ways that don't originate from the core of our being. Without regularly nurturing and taking time to honor that core, we may become alienated from it.

The techniques that best allow us to gain access to our core self vary from person to person. Whatever method we use, we must penetrate through our psychological and emotional layers to a quieter place within, a place of silence that effortlessly generates healing and nurturing.

Getting Motivated

To establish a successful yoga practice, you must understand exactly why you are practicing. Whatever your goal—stress reduction, heightened awareness, greater flexibility—it should be personally meaningful.

Contemplate and then answer in writing the following questions:

1. Do I really want to have a yoga practice?

2. Why? Be specific.

3. What do I expect of the practice?

This exercise can help you clarify your desire to practice and determine how important yoga is to you. Your commitment to practicing must be clear. For example, if your main reason for wanting to practice is to reduce the stress caused by your hectic daily schedule, but your best excuse for not practicing is that you don't have time, you have a problem with internal consistency. With this lack of clarity, you run the risk of unintentionally sabotaging your intentions.

Motivation for practice must be personal. Try this little exercise: Describe in writing how you feel after a good yoga class. Be specific, taking time to identify your thoughts, feelings, and sensations. If your response to classes is generally positive, you can motivate yourself by recalling these benefits.

Some people, however, respond with comments like "I was very sore for the next three days," or "I'm so tight that stretching hurts," or "Some poses are emotionally painful for me." If you have such a response, you are likely to find regular practice more difficult. Yet your body is also likely to be the kind that benefits most from a regular daily practice. Have enough faith in yourself, your teacher, and your body to continue exploring the work. With regular practice, your body (and

Getting your mind together with your body is a little like training a horse: it must be done in easy stages.

ELEANOR CRISWELL

mind) will begin to change more rapidly. Because you are releasing muscular tension on a daily basis, you will soon find that the poses come more easily.

Don't evaluate your practice until you have completed an initial period of commitment—ideally, at least three times per week for a period of one to two months. Once this period is over, skip a week and see how you feel. If you miss your practice, begin again. If your life feels just fine without it, then maybe it is not your time or your path. A personal practice must be a gift to yourself, not a burden.

The brain is the hardest part of the body to adjust in asanas.

B. K. S. IYENGAR

Obstacles to Practice

We often sabotage our practice by making excuses for not doing it. Make a list of your ten best excuses. Try not to censor yourself—just free-associate.

This exercise removes obstacles to practice from the recesses of the mind, where they can seem insurmountable. When your obstacles are listed, you can attend to each one systematically, eventually clearing the path. Perhaps the removal of the obstacles will occur in a day; perhaps it will take months. No matter—the removal itself may need to be your practice for now.

Compare your list with the obstacles described by the *Hatha Yoga Pradipika* and Patanjali's *Yoga Sutra*. According to these ancient texts, the obstacles to practice are lack of interest, doubt, laziness, sensuality, false knowledge, failure to concentrate, pain, despair, unsteadiness of body, sickness, and unsteadiness of respiration. Of these eleven obstacles, only four have to do with the physical body. The rest are psychological, reflecting the connection between body, mind, and spirit. The wisdom and applicability of this ancient list continually astounds me.

How does this list compare to your own? How do these texts suggest you deal with your obstacles? To answer these questions, consult and study the ancient works.

Once you have removed your obstacles, assess how much time you are prepared to commit to yoga. Be as realistic as possible. Make an initial estimate, then deduct 15 percent to allow for overenthusiasm.

If you find yourself saying that you don't really have time, spend a day or two writing down what you do with each 15-minute period of your waking life. In most cases, you will find at least half an hour that might be redesignated for the practice of postures (asana). If you find some time but still cannot commit to using it for yoga, then reexamine your priorities to determine whether regular yoga practice is what you want right now. If it is not, then acknowledge this fact and just practice when you feel like it.

Making a Contract

If you have found some extra time to dedicate to yoga, then you are ready to move on to the next step: making a contract. The contract should be a set of significant but realistic commitments. If the contract is unrealistic, it can become a source of stress and guilt, which are unhealthy and unyogic.

Most of us have been raised to believe that a written agreement represents a deeper commitment than an oral one. The writing of a yoga contract requires us to record on paper not only our intention to practice, but also the specifics: How long will we practice? How many times per week? What time? Where?

If you feel resistant to writing out a contract, try it anyway. Writing it out will deepen your commitment, whereas mental contracts are easily shifted, compromised, or completely forgotten.

Guidelines for Practice

Before beginning your practice, be certain that you understand the following guidelines:

1. Regularity is key. Ideally, practice at the same time each day.

2. Ideally, practice six out of seven days, with the seventh being a day of complete rest. (But if you can't, don't feel guilty. It is better to practice just a little—and enjoy it—than not to practice at all.)

3. Don't eat for two hours before practicing.

4. Practice in a clean, quiet, flat area out of direct sunlight.

5. Don't bounce into a stretch; rather, allow each stretch to develop gradually.

6. Go as far into each pose as you can while maintaining proper alignment.

7. Don't practice with a fever. If weak or tired, do a supportive practice.

8. In each pose, observe the following: How do you feel? How do you respond to the pose? Where do you feel strength, fatigue, weakness, or tightness? Does the pose elicit an emotional response? What does the pose teach you about yourself?

Organizing Your Practice

A balanced practice should have a sense of flow and movement. This flow generally begins with a warm-up and centering phase, gradually makes a transition to a period of increased intensity focusing on a particular category of poses, and culminates in a final stage that cools and quiets the nervous system.

Warm-up and Centering

The warm-up and centering phase is very significant. It helps you realize that your practice of the postures is a separate part of your day, a time to take the energy you normally expend on the world and turn it inward to nurture your body, mind, and soul.

In addition to centering you, this portion of the practice prepares your body by opening the hips, groins, and shoulders. Because certain poses prepare us more effectively for certain types of practices, it is important that you make some basic decisions before starting: What will the major emphasis of my practice be? Will I work with forward-bending or backbending poses? How much time do I have today? Without this decision-making process, practice becomes casual and unfocused. I am not suggesting that there is no room for intuitive practice. I do suggest, however, that you limit how often you work that way. Deep practice, encompassing the physical, emotional, and spiritual dimensions, is more likely to arise from an organized, structured approach.

Having answered these questions, you can use this first phase as a time to open and prepare your whole being for practice. A ritualized beginning is crucial, as it provides structure. If this portion of the practice is handled in a nonfeeling, mindless, remote-control way, then the activity becomes stretching, as opposed to asana. Self-study (svadhyaya) must go on at each moment, to ensure that practice is not limited to the physical level.

Use the centering phase to tune in to and honor what your energy level actually is, rather than coming into the practice with an expectation of what your energy should be and then doing poses to try to shift it. Use this time to determine whether the rest of your practice will be active and vigorous or passive and supported. Be certain that your deci-

If you are out of your body . . . you need a substitute for the feeling of being grounded. Much of what passes for "culture" and "personality" in our society tends to fall into this substitute category, and is in fact the result of running from silence, and from genuine somatic experience.

MORRIS BERMAN

sion results from your body's needs and not from your ego. To practice passively at a time when you need to work more actively is laziness. To practice actively when supported work is more appropriate is violence.

Find a combination of poses that both centers you and prepares your body for the type of practice you have chosen.

In this first phase of practice, the concentration with which we perform the poses moves us closer to our spiritual center. Our personal attraction to particular poses allows us to center more easily in some than in others. Our responsibility as students is to open ourselves to this state in every asana, thus allowing each one to nurture us fully.

Journaling

A final component of establishing a practice is using a journal. Journaling allows you to keep systematic track of the poses and practices you do, and your response to them. A journal should include the date; time of practice; duration of practice; order of postures; postures avoided; feelings and insights; and knowledge gaps. This process will not only help you observe your own growth, but will come in handy if you are having particular problems. For example, if after certain practice sessions you are irritable, referring to your journal will help you systematically determine which poses led you to feel this way. If you still cannot sort it out, take your journal to a skilled teacher who can evaluate your sequencing. Recording classes or workshops in your journal is also helpful.

At the end of each month, write for half an hour about any pose that you choose. Here are some questions to get you started: What is the overall feeling of the pose? What are the specific instructions for doing it? What are some refinements to it? What other poses help you prepare for it? What props might you use to deepen your understanding?

Organizing and establishing a personal practice is by no means a simple or casual process. Obstacles arise each day that can be easily justified as good reasons not to practice. When we submit to these obstacles and lose our motivation, we must call on our self-discipline to assist us. The discipline to practice despite other pressing matters is of key importance.

Whether we approach our daily yoga with energy or reluctance, practice can move us toward a more positive, balanced state. When we act from this state, our interactions with the world are more harmonious. Thus our practice is not only for our own benefit, but is truly a practice for the planet as a whole.

Hatha Yoga plays an important part in the development of a human being. It leads to an exploration of the potential of the body, working in harmony with the mind, to bring the seeker into closer contact with the Higher Self.

SWAMI SIVANANDA RADHA

RESOURCES

Books

Baldwin, C. *Life's Companion: Journal Writing as a Spiritual Quest.* New York: Bantam Books, 1991.

Hunt, D., and P. Hait. *The Tao of Time.* New York: Fireside Books, 1990.

Progoff, I. *At a Journal Workshop.* New York: Dialogue House, 1975. This is the basic text and guide for using the Intensive Journal, a method of keeping a journal for personal growth devised by the American psychotherapist Ira Progoff.

Servan-Schreiber, J.–L. *The Art of Time.* New York: Addison-Wesley, 1988.

Wakefield, D. *The Story of Your Life: Writing a Spiritual Autobiography.* Boston, MA: Beacon Press, 1990.

We have neglected our emotional reality, and the source of our self-nourishment: our bodies.

STANLEY KELEMAN

A NONVIOLENT APPROACH TO EXTENDING YOUR LIMITS
BY KEN DYCHTWALD, PH.D.

The yoga perspective recognizes that each of us is made up of a great many forces, feelings, limits, possibilities, and passions. These aspects exist within my body and my mind and collectively define the boundaries that I usually identify as "me." Physically, these limits are experienced as muscle tension, restricted movement, and pain. Psychologically, limits are experienced as dogma, ignorance, and fear. Most limits have the potential to continually change and restructure themselves.

Now, if I sit on the floor and try to reach over to touch my toes, I might notice that I can only stretch to about five inches away from my toes before I experience tension and slight pain. At this point, the muscles in my lower back and the muscles in the back of my legs are just too tight to allow me any further stretch. At this point I am experiencing one of my boundaries.

This point, this "edge," is a highly important place, for within the yogic philosophy, this edge is considered to be my creative teacher from whom I can learn about myself. If I approach this teacher/edge with love, sensitivity, and awareness, I will discover that my teacher/edge will move and allow me a greater range of motion. If I shy away from approaching my teacher/edge, I will learn nothing new, and in time my own dogma/tightness will contract upon itself and I will grow even tighter.

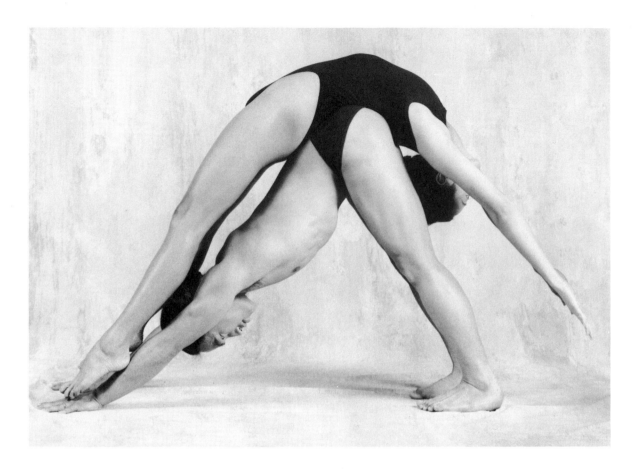

If I try to blast past my edge, I might fool myself into thinking that I have learned and expanded, but in fact what usually happens is that I am only impressing myself with a temporary surge of ambition and that this feeling will probably contract upon itself with fear and subsequent tightening, forcing me into greater confusion or potentially dangerous misunderstandings. Physically, when I approach my edge gently and consciously, my body responds by focusing energy and attention on this spot, encouraging the blood and energy to bathe the related muscles and organs with vitality and life, thus allowing me the experience of true growth and self-nourishment. But if I do not try to reach my edge, my body, having no point of focus, will find it difficult to isolate the place and nourish it, and little growth and improvement will follow.

To state the extremes: If I never explore my limits, my bodymind will gradually tighten and become unconscious. If I regularly explore my limits in a caring and adventuresome fashion, I will expand and grow in a vital fashion. But if I try to push myself past where I am honestly able to go, I will no longer be practicing "yoga" but instead will be practicing "greed," and I will probably be met by pain and disease. Stated simply, it is the difference between ignoring your self, making love to yourself, and raping yourself.

The other fascinating aspect is that the teacher/edge, in addition to defining the limits of expansion and contraction, also distinguishes the fine line that exists between self-destruction and self-improvement. Thus, the artist continually strives to reach deeper past his own abilities and limits in order to experience a new idea, a creative insight, or an illuminating vision. But if he pushes himself past his own limits too fast or too hard, he might experience tension, pain, and suffering. And so will the athlete or yogi who does the same. When psychological or physical growth are pushed too hard, the movement toward expansion and growth is often forced to take a side turn into the domain of pain, stress, and discomfort.

Now, what does all of this have to do with health, dis-ease, and personal growth? Well, the implication of this yogic perspective is that health, dis-ease, and personal growth are all aspects of the way in which you deal with yourself. When you are being loving to yourself and are without chronically painful conflicts, your bodymind will manifest a state of health. Similarly, when you are being unconscious and unloving toward yourself, you run the risk of moving your bodymind into a state of dis-ease and stress, which could undermine your health and hamper your growth.

This perspective also suggests that the most effective and efficient way to develop yourself is to be as mindful and as aware as possible, all the while being respectful of self-limits and appreciative of continually regenerating expansiveness.

This perspective reflects the yogic nonviolent, noncompetitive, holistic approach to growth, education, and health, in contrast to our Western philosophy and health practices, which are often competitive, aggressive, and self-insensitive.

WORKING WITH THE BREATH
BY RICHARD C. MILLER, PH.D.

To see the importance of breathing in relation to other physiological "intake" activities, consider that although we may drink as much as a few quarts of water and eat as much as a few pounds of food each day,

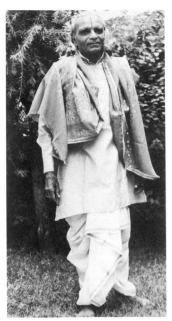

B. K. S. IYENGAR

we breathe roughly 23,000 times daily and take in about 12,000 liters (4,500 gallons) of air—and 25 times that amount during exercise! No wonder the way we breathe profoundly influences the health of our body and mind.

Breath and Movement

Our physical existence depends upon breath. Breathing plays a fundamental role in our every activity and is critical in all the physiological functions of the human body. But breathing is not merely a physical process; it is also closely connected with the functioning of the mind and emotions. When we are upset, agitated, depressed, or even excessively happy, our breathing patterns change. When our breathing rhythms are altered, our state of mind and emotions are affected, and repressed feelings, thoughts, and emotions may be released. Conversely, if we regularize our breathing rhythms, our thoughts and emotions stabilize, allowing us to become more relaxed and at ease.

Movement and Breath

Breathing directly affects both external and internal movement and is one of the most efficient ways of influencing the shape of the spine, the single most important structure in the practice of hatha yoga. The forces generated during physical movement tend to originate in the exterior muscles and travel inward toward the spine and the deeper regions of the body. The movement that occurs during deep breathing, by contrast, begins in the deeper regions of the body near the spine and travels outward toward the exterior. This outward movement occurs as a function of the way in which the muscles of respiration are attached deep in the body. By synchronizing all physical movements with the breath, therefore, we can gain both internal and external benefits. Such synchronization maximizes the effect of the movements on the spinal column, the visceral tissues and organs, and the external muscles.

Try the movements described in Figure 1 and observe how the breath helps or hinders your performance.

We can now formulate some general guidelines for breathing during movement:

1. Forward bending occurs most easily during exhalation.

2. Backward bending is generally executed during inhalation.

3. Twisting movements occur most readily during exhalation.

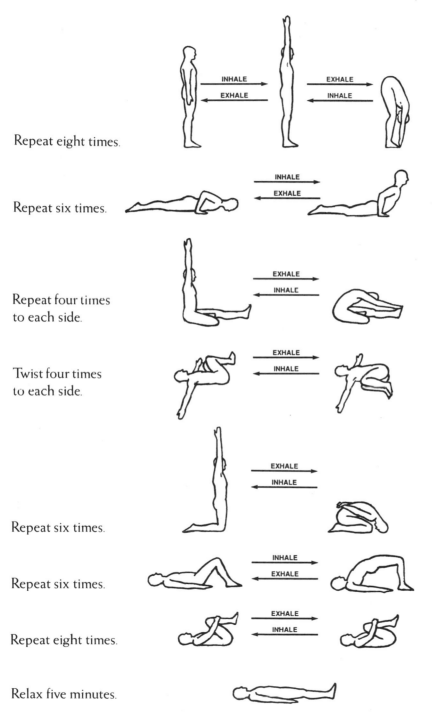

Repeat eight times.

Repeat six times.

Repeat four times
to each side.

Twist four times
to each side.

Repeat six times.

Repeat six times.

Repeat eight times.

Relax five minutes.

FIGURE ONE
All movements are repeated in a dynamic manner: Move back and forth in the same posture while breathing. Take a long, deep exhalation and a long, deep inhalation.

4. Movements that expand the chest and thorax are initiated during inhalation.

5. Movements that compress the abdominal area and thorax region are initiated during exhalation.

Qualities of the Breath

The breath is a powerful ally in our practice and is to be respected as a vital component of every movement we make. In the *Yoga Sutra*, Patanjali places special emphasis on the correct use of the breath, considering it an important indicator of the state of one's body and mind, as well as a means for clarifying the mind and promoting greater awareness. Patanjali suggests that the breath be long, comfortable, and refined. He also recommends the practice of exhalation and mild retention after exhalation as a means toward that end.

When we work with our breath, its motion should take on the beautiful, rhythmic shape of a sine wave. Notice that the exhalation is longer than the inhalation. This is because for the average person the normal exhalation is about one and one-half times as long as the inhalation. During asana practice we adjust the exhalation to this ratio and try to stabilize this breathing pattern throughout the practice. For example, if your inhalation is six seconds long, extend your exhalation to nine seconds. Some students need to develop their ability to inhale, whereas others need to learn how to exhale more fully. Eventually, however, the ratio should approach 1:1.5 during asana practice. We may, of course, decide to alter this ratio, depending on what effect we wish to achieve.

In hatha yoga, we do not consciously strive for quantity, volume, or depth of air in the lungs, because such efforts ultimately result in sacrificing the quality of the breath. Instead, greater quantity and depth result naturally from the control and smoothness we develop in our breathing.

Begin with Exhalation

Traditionally, we teach students how to exhale when they are learning to synchronize the breath in movement. It is safer to exhale in any movement, and the body feels looser and more capable of movement during the exhalation. Exhalation tends to promote a relaxation response, whereas inhalation may make a person feel tense or constricted. Inhalation occurs automatically and develops spontaneously as the exhalation becomes refined and smooth.

Hatha Yoga is based on the principle that changes in consciousness can be brought about by setting in motion currents of certain kinds of subtler forces in the physical body.

I. K. TAIMNI

The mind is connected with the life force indwelling in all beings. Like a bird tied to a string: so is the mind.

The mind is not brought under control by many considerations. The means for its control is nothing else but the life force.

GORAKSHA PADDHATI

Exhalation should never be forced, but should be slow and comfortable. The yogic breathing technique of *ujjayi* (constriction of the throat) is recommended, because it brings a sense of control as well as a sound to which we may listen as we learn to measure and become aware of the breath. Ujjayi breathing also promotes an easy feeling in the body. [This technique is performed by slightly constricting the throat, which produces a mild snoring noise during inhalation and exhalation.—Eds.]

As we begin to synchronize the movements of the body with the flow of the breath, we learn to respect the feedback we gain from listening to the breath. Notice that as the body fatigues, the breath becomes rough and unruly, indicating the need for a rest or change in posture. Also, observe that when we are no longer able to maintain evenness in the breath during a practice session (no matter how long we rest between postures or how simple a variation we choose), it is time to end our practice for that day. The sound and texture of the breath also gives us indications of impending colds or other illnesses, providing advance warning so that we may take steps to avoid the disease before it develops. There are many yogic techniques for using the breath to prevent or heal diseases.

Breath Surrounds the Posture

Beginning students tend either to hold the breath as they move or to begin their movements before they begin to breathe. Instead, the breath should "surround" all movements in asana (Figure 1). Try practicing the movements in Figure 2 by beginning your breath just slightly before you begin to move in the postures and ending your breath just slightly after you end the movements. During this practice, all movements should be completely synchronized with the inhalation and exhalation. As an extreme example, even if you are only moving your little finger up and down, synchronize the breath with each of the movements. When the breath is consciously used in this manner, the mind remains focused.

The Stillness Between Inhalation and Exhalation

Observe your breathing patterns right now. You may notice that your inhalation and exhalation are fairly regular, but shallow. Also, observe the slight hesitation between each breath. This naturally occurring hesitation is similar to the pause that occurs when the pendulum of a clock reaches the top of its arc. There is a moment of stillness before it

Prana is in the air, but is not the oxygen, nor any of its chemical constituents. It is in food, water, and in the sunlight, yet it is not vitamin, heat, or light-rays. Food, water, air, etc. are only the media through which the prana is carried.

SWAMI VISHNUDEVANANDA

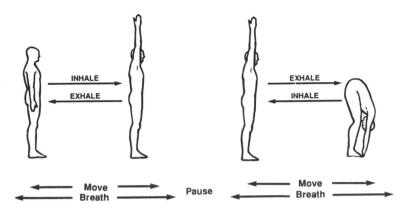

FIGURE TWO

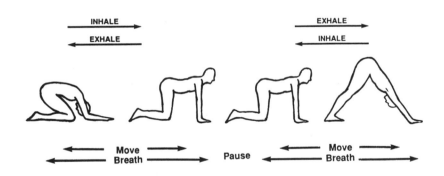

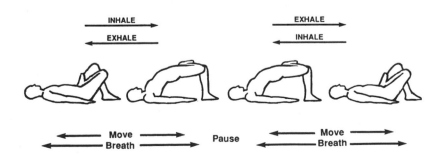

descends into the next phase of its movement.

Once you can synchronize your inhalation and exhalation with each of your movements, turn your attention to the hesitation between each breath and experiment with the length of this pause. Observe that each of your breaths tends to run right into the next one and that the pause between breaths is barely noticeable. (We are concerned here with a pause of perhaps one to two seconds. Later, we will discuss holding the breath for longer periods of time.)

The pause between breaths is very important. This pause is a moment of meditative stillness in which we have an opportunity to see ourselves clearly. Notice that as you practice, your mind tends to wander from the task at hand. You may suddenly find yourself reviewing a past or future event that is totally unrelated to your present activity. The mind needs constant attention. Each time it wanders away, bring it back tenaciously to your present activity. One goal of yoga is to be able to hold the mind focused for as long as it takes to achieve our purpose. Pausing after each breath helps us to achieve this goal. The pause has a centering effect on the mind, keeping us focused on what we are doing and serving as a reminder for us to bring the mind back from its wanderings.

Also, become aware of the stillness that pervades the pause. When you come back to movement following each pause, bring this stillness with you. Then all movement will be seen to arise out of stillness, unfold in stillness, and disappear back into stillness. Movement done in this manner unfolds without effort, tension, or expectation and continually refers us back to the stillness which is our real nature.

At the end of each breath (and consequently at the end of each movement), try adding a short pause of one to two seconds in length. During the pause, suspend all movement in your body and breath and become absolutely still. In this stillness you will have an opportunity to observe the quality of your mind as well as the stillness that lies beyond the mind.

Yoga is a science of being awareness, and hatha yoga is one tool we may use to uncover this eternal truth. The pause between breaths reminds us to observe ourselves during our practice so that we may investigate whether we are using the mind and breath or they are using us.

The Dynamics of Natural Forces in the Body

We must learn to appreciate the forces that arise within the body in response to the breath during asana and breath control (pranayama). We

Breath is the physical counterpart of the mind.

HARISH JOHARI

Breathing, then, is intercourse
with the universe, with all of life.

JUNE SINGER

have previously mentioned the conflicting forces that arise when the body's external movements are contrary to the forces created by the breath, as occurs when we attempt to initiate forward bends during inhalation. Now consider the forces that arise in the body as you practice inhaling and exhaling during movement.

The natural forces created by forward bending (and twisting) movements begin in the lower spine and travel upward toward the neck. Similarly, the natural forces that occur during exhalation move from the lower spine upward toward the neck. Natural forces that arise during backbending begin in the upper body (thorax and chest) and travel downward toward the sacrum. Likewise, the natural forces that occur during inhalation begin in the chest and move downward toward the diaphragm.

When the inhalation and exhalation are properly performed in this manner, the spine extends with each breath. As we inhale, the action of the breath inside the body, along with the action of the intercostal (rib) and other supporting muscles, provides a downward-moving force that actually lifts and extends the vertebral column as if it were being pulled up from the top. When we exhale, the action of the breath inside the body, together with the action of the abdominal muscles and diaphragm, provides an upward-moving force that stabilizes the spine and supports the lifting and extension that occurred during inhalation. Thus, correctly synchronizing the breath with movements in the postures gives us a superb way to create extension in the spine, allowing us to derive maximum benefit from our practice with the most efficient expenditure of energy.

Movement Influences Breath

Just as the breath influences bodily movement, so bodily movement influences the breath. We must respect this relationship between movement and breath and learn to utilize its beneficial aspects when choosing asanas, sequences of asanas, and breathing ratios.

It is important not to allow movements to disturb the breath. One challenge of hatha yoga is to become proficient at handling increasingly greater amounts of "resistance" (complexity and degree of difficulty) in the various postures and breathing patterns while maintaining a steady and comfortable equilibrium of body and mind. We can create such resistance by changing either the posture, the posture variation, or the breathing ratio with which we work. In the final analysis, however, it is our ability to maintain a smooth, stable quality of the breath that will determine the stability and comfort we achieve in our practice. Because of the relationship that exists between mind, breath, and body, it is far easier to still the body than to still the breath. If the mind is disturbed, the breath becomes disturbed long before the body.

It is more effective to measure the amount of time you spend in a pose by counting the number of breaths, rather than by counting the number of seconds or minutes elapsed. Measuring the number and quality of breaths gives you a more effective gauge of determining your stamina of mind and body and prevents the practice from becoming goal- or externally oriented.

Vinyasa Krama

Up to this point, we have assumed that each breath is long, smooth, and continuous, and that there is a brief pause after each breath. There is another way of breathing in movement that brings a new effect to our practice. It is called *krama* in Sanskrit, meaning "to proceed in intelligently conceived steps in order to reach a desired goal." In krama, movements are linked to the breath in a series of distinct steps, or stages, thus allowing us to challenge our stamina in movement or our ability to maintain a steady and harmonious breath while under increased resistance.

We may work with linking breath and movement which emphasizes one's ability to move the body in distinct stages while controlling the breath in unison with the movements. Or we may work with staging the breath while keeping a fixed pose.

Depending on the variation we choose, our physical work may be increased or decreased, adding or subtracting difficulty from the task of maintaining a steady and comfortable breath. We may challenge ourselves infinitely by choosing a multiple of variations within the same pose, as well as by varying the number of pauses during each breath.

Why should one vary one's practice in this way? We may wish to add a new dimension to our stamina or ability to concentrate; we may be interested in bringing attention to a certain area of the body or to one aspect of the breath; we may wish to accentuate the effect of posture or breath on the mind; or we may wish to add variety to our usual practice to create innovation and new learning.

Become proficient in the "normal" ways of regulating the poses and breath before attempting vinyasa krama. Otherwise, you may overstrain your body and breath and become mentally agitated.

Holding the Breath

There is a difference between pausing between breaths and holding the breath. Holding the breath involves a longer duration and introduces a new element of synchronizing breath and movement in asana. Given the previously discussed rules for breathing, it follows that holding the breath after an inhalation should occur when the body is in extension, whereas holding after an exhalation may occur during either extension or flexion of the body.

Initially, you will want to investigate holding the breath when you are not moving your body. Eventually you will want to explore holding your breath while moving your body.

When holding the breath, all of the previously discussed rules of breathing apply. You should keep the breath and the movement under your control, and you should remain comfortable and steady throughout the process. It is not helpful to hold the breath only to become winded and fatigued when you start to breathe again. This is not the desired effect. Patanjali has set forth a number of symptoms to watch for when practicing yoga which signal the presence of an obstacle that will interfere with your mental clarity. These symptoms are: mental discomfort, negative thinking, inability to remain at ease in your posture, and difficulty in regulating your breath. Holding the breath too long may produce these symptoms and prevent you from obtaining your desired goal. So proceed carefully when first experimenting with holding the breath during movement.

Visualization

Once we have mastered the techniques and principles of breathing and integrated them into our practice, we can combine them in different ways to produce myriad effects on our body and mind. We must take the time, however, to fully appreciate the subtlety of each technique. There is more to breathing than may first meet the eye, as illustrated by a story concerning the first meeting between Gurdjieff and his Sufi teacher. When the teacher asked him the purpose of his visit, Gurdjieff is said to have replied, "I just want to learn how to breathe," a reply that elicited peals of laughter from the Sufi, who went on to spend many years teaching Gurdjieff "just how to breathe."

Visualization can play an important role in learning the art of synchronizing breath and movement. You can visualize how a movement will look when practiced with a continuous and harmonious breath.

Then you can physically attempt the movement, making further refinements in your visualization, movement, and breathing as you proceed.

Another approach involves visualizing and feeling the movement of the breath inside your body. As you exhale, visualize the breath moving upward along your spine from the coccyx to the crown. Reverse the visualization on the inhalation, imaginging the breath descending from the crown to the base of the spine. Similarly, practice visualizing and feeling how the forces in the body flow from the base to the crown of the spine on flexion and from the crown to the base of the spine in extension. Then, synchronize these two movements so that, as you exhale and flex the body, you feel the upward movement of the breath harmonizing with the flow of movements in the posture, and as you inhale and extend the body, you feel the downward movement of the breath harmonizing with the downward movements of the posture.

You can also visualize and feel the movement of your diaphragm as you breathe and move. As you inhale, the diaphragm descends, pushing gently on the abdominal wall and increasing the internal pressure in the abdomen. As you exhale, the diaphragm ascends, causing the abdominal wall to move inward.

As you breathe in a sitting or standing posture, begin to feel this diaphragmatic movement. It is subtle and requires practice. Once you have a sense of how the diaphragm and abdominal muscles work together as a team during inhalation and exhalation, progressively introduce more and more complex movements into your practice, integrating the breath and body movements with your visual images. In this way you will systematically train your mind, body, and breath to work harmoniously together.

Still another way to begin working with breath and movement is to practice a series of forward bends with long exhalations, observing the effects on your mind and body. Then practice a series of backbends with long inhalations, again observing the results. Keep a diary of your observations. Next, try to reverse the breathing in the movements. For example, now do the backbends with long exhalations and note the difference in how you feel after you have finished.

Working in these ways keeps your practice fresh and interesting. It teaches you skills of observation and reflection and sharpens your discipline and willpower. Keeping an ongoing journal will help you learn how the various combinations of breathing and movement affect your body and mind. Thus you will slowly acquire a practical understanding of the principles of breath and movement that have been recorded for thousands of years in the ancient texts of yoga.

Developing a sensitivity to the breath can help us experience a greater sense of space within ourselves. We may then feel more expanded and demand less space around us. Breathing can teach us how to handle our emotions and gain an understanding of our thoughts, thus helping to make our lives more creative, spontaneous, and happy. And, although we may not be fond of discipline, we should remember that the word *discipline* and *disciple* both come from the root meaning "to learn." If we are willing to become disciples of the breath, we will find it to be a very valuable friend and teacher.

RESOURCES

Books

Iyengar, B. K. S. *Light on Pranayama*. New York: Crossroad Publishing, 1981.

Johari, H. *Breath, Mind, and Consciousness*. Rochester, VT: Destiny Books, 1989.

Swami Rama, R. Ballentine, and A. Hymes, *Science of Breath: A Practical Guide*. Honesdale, PA: Himalayan International Institute, 1979.

BREATH AND PRANA

The mind is connected with the life force indwelling in all beings. Like a bird tied to a string: so is the mind.

The mind is not brought under control by many considerations. The means for its control is nothing else but the life force.

This passage can be found in the *Yoga Shikha Upanishad*, which is a medieval Sanskrit scripture on yoga. It makes a most important point, namely that the mind is dependent on what is called *prana*, the life force. This is considered to be a universal and indestructible energy that underlies all things. It is what animates our bodies and what keeps our minds in perpetual motion. The breath is the external or material aspect of that cosmic force.

Another more subtle aspect of prana is the human aura, the multicolored energy field surrounding the physical body, which has been captured in part by Kirlian photography. Sensitives can see the aura, which contains important clues about a person's physical, emotional, and mental well-being.

For thousands of years, the adepts of yoga have known about prana and its various operations in the human body-mind. They discovered that by controlling the breath, they can not only control the mind but also manipulate the flow of prana in and around the body.

Advanced yogic practice, in meditation and visualization, focuses on working with the body's energy field. Anticipating modern physics by several millennia, the yogis claim that, ultimately, the human body-mind is pure light. Thus the yogic discipline of pranayama involves much more than the control of the breath. It is a powerful means of discovering the energetic nature of existence.

RESOURCES

Books

Aivanhov, O. M. *Life Force*. Frejus, France: Prosveta, 1987. A collection of talks by a respected spiritual teacher.

Davidson, J. *Subtle Energy*. Saffron Walden, England: C. W. Daniel Co., 1987. A consideration of subtle forms of energy, including prana.

Karagulla, S., and D. van Gelder Kunz. *The Chakras and the Human Energy Field*. Wheaton, IL: Quest Books, 1989. A collaborative effort between a psychiatrist and a clairvoyant.

Kilner, W. J. *The Aura*. New York: Weiser, 1974. A classic study of the aura, utilizing mechanical means rather than clairvoyance.

Kunz, D. van Gelder. *The Personal Aura*. Wheaton, IL: Quest Books, 1991. This illustrated volume is based on the clairvoyant descriptions of the author. The large color plates give one an excellent sense of what a clairvoyant might see when looking at the aura of healthy and sick individuals.

Note

[1]Sri Aurobindo, *The Life Divine* (Pondicherry, India: Sri Aurobindo Ashram, 1977), pp. 907–908.

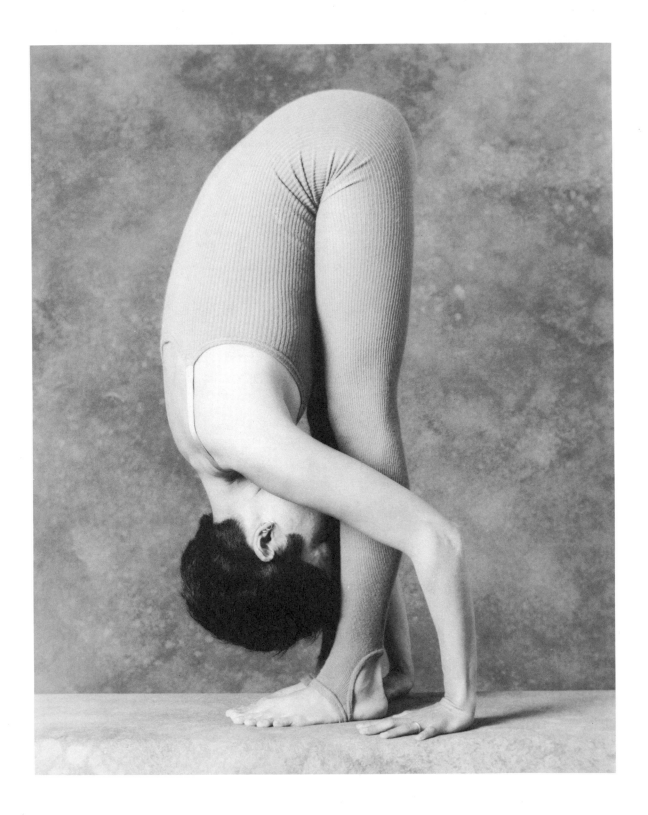

THREE

Yoga Postures and Poise

If you have studied the previous chapter carefully, you will be equipped with its sound advice and can now begin to experiment with the exercises given in the present chapter. Here you will learn how to practice the yogic postures (asanas) correctly, efficiently, and elegantly. These postures are more than they seem to be, because they yield their secret only when they are executed with the right inner disposition.

Another very important aspect of asana practice is sequencing, and we have included an excellent essay to answer all your questions about how to structure your own exercise program. You will be introduced to balancing exercises, forward bends, backward bends, twists, and special exercises for opening up the groin, which, among other things, will help you master the coveted lotus posture. But proceed without hurry, and put your trust in regular discipline rather than speed. Wisdom, including the wisdom of the body, takes time to manifest.

In my own belief there is a divine source of awareness of which the individual lived body partakes, but which it does not exhaust.

DREW LEDER

POSTURE, POSTURING, AND POISE

Our posture says a lot about our inner life. If we appear hunched over, it is probably because we are inwardly collapsed. If we strut about with our chest sticking out and nose in the air, we are undoubtedly posturing, parading our inflated sense of self. Our bearing and our gestures contain valuable clues about our emotional state—it is hard to lie with the body.

Whereas posturing is always an attempt to conceal a weakness, good posture suggests inner balance. When good posture is maintained with ease in all circumstances, we have poise.

The Yoga postures, or asanas, help us achieve not only good posture but also poise. They exercise our muscles, tendons, and organs, and realign our bony frame to function with optimum efficiency by allowing the life force (prana) to flow freely in our whole body. A healthy, radiant body makes it easier to connect with the larger Reality, which nourishes us spiritually. Because the yoga postures are so much more than mere physical exercises, they also cultivate poise, helping us to face all situations bravely and with dignity.

Your whole being should be symmetrical. Yoga is symmetry. That is why Yoga is a basic art.

B. K. S. IYENGAR

RESOURCES

Books

Criswell, E. *How Yoga Works: An Introduction to Somatic Yoga.* Novato, CA: Freeperson Press, 1989.

Iyengar, B. K. S. *Light on Yoga.* New York: Schocken Books, 1966.

Keleman, S. *Your Body Speaks Its Mind.* Berkeley, CA: Center Press, 1981.

Swami Sivananda Radha. *Hatha Yoga: The Hidden Language—Symbols, Secrets, and Metaphor.* Porthill, ID: Timeless Books, 1987.

Swami Vishnudevananda. *The Complete Illustrated Book of Yoga.* New York: Bell Publishing, 1960.

ASANA: BASIC MOVEMENT TOWARD HEALTH
BY JUDITH LASATER, PH.D.

What Is Asana?

Almost all systems of self-transformation begin with the body, whether they are philosophically Eastern or Western in history or orientation. Every meditation system begins with a special position of the body, like the familiar lotus position. This is quickly followed by attention to breathing. Even classical psychoanalysis begun by Sigmund Freud originally had the patient lie down, thus changing mental states by changing physical ones. Asana is merely a special body position which can allow and create special mental effects and changes. Additionally, there are added physiological benefits, some of which will be discussed later.

Another reason the practice of asana, or yogic posture, can be a powerful transformational tool is its nonverbal nature. While practicing asana the student is using the right hemisphere of the brain, the one concerned with movement, the perception of the wholeness of patterns and spatial relationships, not words. Words generally divide thought, and it is this discriminative ability that gives words power. But that very ability to divide can divide us from ourselves, from our bodies and from our emotions. Because the asana is a nonverbal experience, there is not a filter of words between the student and the experience.

Asana thus brings us completely into the present moment. With the practice of asana we become aware of what is, of what sensations exist right now in the body and the corresponding thoughts that exist in the mind. This becoming aware of what is puts us in touch with emotions that may have been ignored or denied. When we are stretching the leg with awareness, that sensation of stretching brings us into the present moment. This coming into the present moment over and over again with the practice of asana, either in a class or at home, creates a habit of awareness. This cognitive habit is meditative and can be emotionally therapeutic.

Posture should be steady and comfortable.

YOGA SUTRA

Tremendous emotional energy is expended because we are ignorant of, or afraid of and therefore denying, what we feel at any moment. The sensation of stretching and opening is the focus of the asana, unlike most of our waking moments when we are expected to ignore our physical sensations. The wonderful paradox of awareness is that when we become truly aware of what is, things begin to change. All other approaches to sensation are forms of running away. For no other reason than this, asana practice can be a wonderful antidote to the stress of modern life.

Asana can be defined as physical positioning that coordinates breathing with moving and holding still for the purpose of both stretching and strengthening parts of the body. In addition, the movements close and squeeze and then open and soak internal organs with blood and nourishment, leading to a deep state of rest and health. *The three basic movements of asana are backbends, forward bends and twisting movements.* These three will be discussed separately, and a simple example of each movement will be given.

Backbends

During normal daily life the vertebral column is often placed in a position of flexion, or slight rounding forward. Check your position as you read this article. Probably you are sitting or lying in a manner that drops the chin toward the chest, thus flexing the cervical spine, as well as rounding the lower back while sitting in a chair or on the bed. There is nothing intrinsically wrong with this position for the cervical and lumbar spines; the problem is that this position of flexion is held too long and too often, thus habitually distorting the normal curves of these areas.

This constant distortion of these two important curves of the neck and lower back put strain on the soft tissues of the area, such as ligaments (which hold bone to bone), tendons (which hold muscles to bone), and the muscles themselves. Feel the muscles at the top of your shoulders; most people feel a deep hardness and tension there. This is evidence of the tension the soft tissue or muscle is maintaining. When normal daily posture becomes habitually out of alignment, strain is produced. For most people in Western culture, this habitual pattern of standing and sitting is a flexed one. For this reason, backbending asanas are beneficial for most yoga students. In addition to restoring the normal status of the cervical and lumbar curves, the movement into a backbend and the holding of this position against gravity strengthens the posterior (back) muscles. This strength can give better support to the column during normal daily life.

Backbending also opens up the chest and can have respiratory benefits for those students whose chest tends to be closed and who may have breathing difficulties. Backbends gently stress the bones of the back because the muscles attached to the vertebrae pull on those vertebrae during the practice of the posture. This stress stimulates the bones to maintain calcium in their structure. This contributes to a healthy skeleton, especially in post-menopausal women, who tend to lose bone mass due to hormonal changes.

To practice a simple backbend, lie on your abdomen on a comfortable surface like a thick rug or a blanket. Rest the head on the forehead. Stretch the arms out to the side so that the body is in the shape of the letter T. Place the legs about hip width apart. Prepare by breathing in and out normally for a couple of breaths. On an exhalation, stretch the arms out and lift the body up, keeping the legs and pelvis on the floor. The arms should be no higher than the shoulders, the back is arched, and the chest is lifted. Continue to breath normally. Hold the pose for several breaths before coming back down to the floor. Refresh yourself with a couple of easy breaths. Repeat the posture. More advanced practitioners can hold the pose longer and repeat it more than twice.

At no time during the posture should there be any discomfort in the lower back; any sensation that is felt there should be that of muscles working, nothing more. Many people report that backbends give them a feeling of energy and aliveness. One theory for this is that the back-bending movement compresses the kidney-adrenal area. When the asana is finished, it is believed that the area is then soaked with blood and that this alternate squeezing and flushing of tissues with blood contributes to the healthy functioning of these organs.

This simple backbend is a variation of a classic yoga asana called the Cobra Pose. It is strengthening for all the muscles on the posterior or back part of the body. This asana is especially good for strengthening the muscles between the scapulae (shoulder blades). These muscles help keep the scapulae in a good position in relationship to the backbone during standing. In addition, this posture strengthens the erector muscles which run parallel to the vertebral column and which help to maintain the normal curve in the lumbar spine. These muscles are stretched during sitting.

Twists

Another major category of yoga asanas is twisting postures. This type of movement alternately stretches and strengthens the lateral muscles of the trunk and can be used for gentle abdominal strengthening as well. In addition, twisting motions compress the abdominal organs such as the intestines, and this alternating pressure seems to aid in their function. Any twisting motion strongly affects the intervertebral discs, which are fibro-cartilaginous pads that are found between most moving vertebrae. What is significant about these pads is that they receive no direct blood supply after the third decade of life. It is important for these discs to be full of fluid to keep the vertebrae apart. If the discs become dried out, thus allowing the vertebrae to approximate (grow nearer), two undesirable things could occur. The disc itself could move or bulge out of place. This in turn could press on one of the spinal nerves, causing pain and possible muscle and sensory impairment.

Twisting asanas actually compress the disc. When the twist is released, the disc then takes up fluid from the surrounding tissues in a process called imbibition. This process, which helps the disc to remain full and plump, is akin to alternately squeezing a sponge and releasing it. One of the hallmarks of yoga asana practice is that the posture should be performed as similarly as possible on both sides of the body. Therefore the discs receive the benefit of compression and release evenly on both sides of the body.

To practice a simple twist, lie down on a comfortable surface.

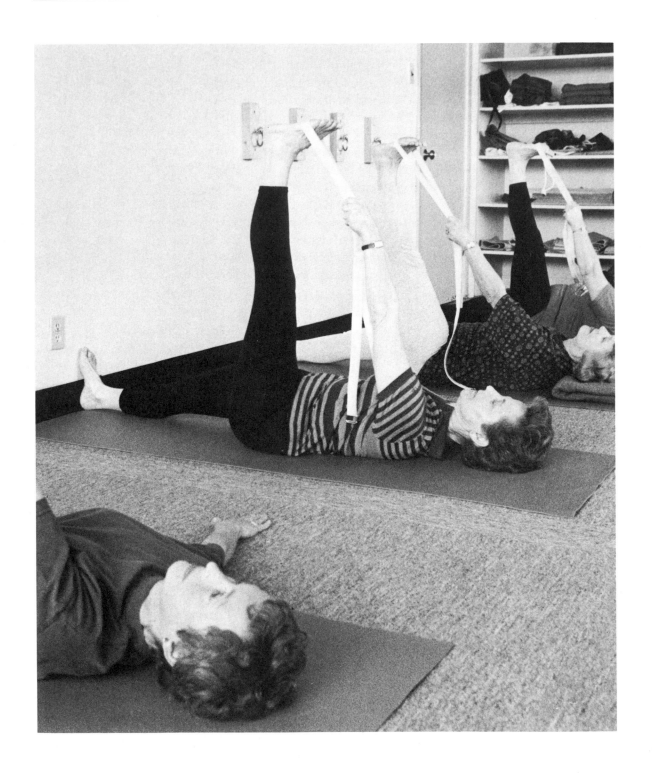

Stretch the arms out to the side of the body to form the same "T" shape that was explained in the backbend instructions given above. With an exhalation, bend the right knee toward the chest and then roll onto the left side so that the right knee comes near to or on the floor. Attempt to keep the right shoulder on the floor while stretching out the right arm. This stretch of the right arm in the opposite direction as the right leg gives a pleasant sensation of stretch along the entire right trunk and sometimes even in the area of the right chest. Turn the head and look at the right hand. Breathe several normal breaths. Slowly return to the back. Straighten out the right leg. Rest a moment and repeat by bending the left knee to the chest and rolling on the right side. After a few breaths return to the back. This posture can be varied by changing the position of the knee relative to the chest. Many students enjoy following this twist by bringing both knees to the chest for a moment. Repeat this posture two or three times as desired. This asana feels particularly good if the back is sore or if one has been standing a lot during the day. It can be practiced after the backbend given previously.

Forward Bends

The final major category of yoga asana movements is forward bending. Forward bends are usually difficult for most adults and for many children because of the tightness of an important set of muscles. These muscles are the hamstring muscles; they begin at the back of the pelvis and thigh, travel down the thigh, and insert on both sides of the knee. They govern the bending of the knee and the extension of the hip joint. Most athletic activities tend to tighten the hamstring muscles and make bending forward difficult. This occurs especially in those who run frequently. When one is running, the hamstring muscles act to decelerate the thigh as it moves forward with great momentum. This deceleration causes the hamstrings to contract strongly with every running step and thereby become tighter and tighter. Unfortunately, the hamstrings can become tighter from inactivity as well, because sitting does not stretch them either.

Most beginning yoga students have tight hamstrings; in fact, so do most intermediate students. A safe yet effective stretch for the hamstrings is one that is done standing. Too often when beginners attempt to stretch the hamstrings from a seated forward bend what actually bends is the middle and lower spines. This reverses the lumbar curve, a position we are all too likely to assume habitually during the day.

In order to stretch the hamstrings effectively and at the same time

As an asana is perfected through practice, at a certain stage it becomes spiritual, a mudra. *The word* mudra *means "a seal, a sealing posture." The royal houses and nobility use seals to signify their position and authenticity. In ancient times the seal was the confirmation of the sender of a message. The human body is also a seal. We have to discover what is sealed up, what is the secret behind the seal.*

SWAMI SIVANANDA RADHA

save the back, try this simple stretch. Stand near a stairway so that the bannister can be used for balance. Place one foot onto a step so that it is about two feet high. The supporting foot should face straight toward the steps and not turn out. The kneecap of the upper leg should face straight up toward the ceiling. The most crucial part of the alignment of the pose concerns the pelvis. Most students will easily bend forward from the waist in this position, but this is not what is effective and safe as a hamstring stretch.

In each pose there should be repose.

B. K. S. IYENGAR

Keeping one hand on the bannister for balance, place the other hand on the rim of the pelvis, just about the level of the navel and at the side. You should feel a bony rim under your thumb and index fingers. This rim should tilt forward when one stretches forward. If this pelvic rim is not moving, then it is probable that the forward movement is coming from the spinal column and not from the pelvis moving forward on the hip joints. Even very supple individuals will feel a stretch in the hamstrings at the back of the thigh if this movement is practiced correctly. Try imagining that the tailbone is tipping up in the back. Notice that very little movement is experienced and yet there is a lot of stretch felt in the hamstrings. If the movement is large, chances are that it is being done incorrectly. Hold the stretch for several breaths and then repeat it on the other side. More advanced pupils should attempt to put the leg higher, but remember that even supple people can feel the stretch with the leg at a fairly low level.

During these asanas, attention is brought first to the area of the body being stretched or contracted, then to the sensation itself, then to the breath, and finally, if appropriate, to the mental reaction to that stretch. This progressive turning inward toward sensation is a focusing technique that yogic asanas provide through the mechanism of stretching. Asana is a straightforward and practical technique that makes concrete the process of becoming present in the moment. Through this process one can surrender the old patterns of feeling and being and move toward the freshness of the possible.

SECRETS OF SEQUENCING
BY DONALD MOYER

Planning your practice. Students who want to begin a yoga practice at home frequently ask how long and how often they should practice. Fifteen to twenty minutes two or three times a week is an adequate start. What matters most is regularity and consistency. I suggest that you make a chart of your weekly routines, such as work and other commitments. Do you have time to practice in the morning or evening, and how much time can you realistically set aside? Let yoga be a welcome and an integral part of your life, not merely another chore or obligation. The following guidelines are intended to help you develop your practice, and to give you some idea of how to choose and sequence postures. The three sample routines included here cover all the basic postures and take approximately forty-five minutes to an hour each to complete.

Eating. The postures (asanas) should be practiced on an empty stomach. Therefore, it is best not to eat for at least two hours prior to your yoga session. If this is not possible to arrange, you may have a light snack (fruit, yogurt) at least an hour before.

Clothing. Wear loose clothing that does not constrict the movement of the pelvis and legs. Practice with bare feet so that you develop sensitivity and strength in the feet and also avoid slipping.

Practice environment. If possible, choose a warm, quiet place to practice where you will not be disturbed. (Turn on your answering machine or unplug your telephone before you begin your session.) A room with a plain wooden floor and a bare wall is ideal. If the only available practice space has a plushy carpet or slippery surface, use a non-slip mat for your standing postures. You will find suitable yoga mats ("sticky mats") advertised in *Yoga Journal.*

Sunshine. If you are practicing outdoors, do not practice directly in the sun, particularly inverted postures. Likewise do not begin a yoga session immediately after you have been out in the hot sun.

Props. Besides a sticky mat, the other props you may need for your yoga practice include:

- a long strap about six feet in length (for use in leg stretches and sitting postures if your hamstrings are tight)

- a wooden block ($3'' \times 5'' \times 9''$) or a stack of books (for support in the standing postures)

- a face cloth or hand towel (for making a knee roll or neck roll)

- a belt with a buckle (for bracing your arms in Shoulderstand and Handstand)

- a single blanket for sitting postures and relaxation

- a pile of blankets about four inches high (for practicing Shoulderstand)

■ a folding or straight-backed chair, with a flat seat rather than a contoured seat

Sequencing your practice. Think of your yoga session as having three distinct phases—a beginning, a middle, and an end. This will help you organize your practice in a harmonious and logical sequence, so that you derive maximum benefit from the postures and avoid injury.

Begin your practice with two or three postures that help to warm up the body and relieve initial stiffness. In this section of your practice you might include the following postures: Adhomukha Shvanasana (Downward-facing Dog Pose), Leg Stretches, or Surya Namaskara (Sun Salutation).

Once you have warmed the body by stretching the arms, the legs, and the spine, you are ready to move to the core of your practice. This section may include standing postures, which develop the strength of the legs, or backbends and twists, which require more suppleness in the spine.

After the dynamic part of your routine, it is time for postures that are more soothing for the nerves, such as Sarvangasana (Shoulderstand), sitting forward bends, or postures in the supine position. Always conclude your practice with several minutes of Shavasana (Corpse Pose), so that you leave your session renewed and refreshed.

Time of day. Whether you practice in the morning, afternoon, or evening makes a considerable difference in how you begin your yoga session.

If you practice in the late afternoon, after a stressful day at work, you may need to begin with some restful postures, such as lying on your back with your feet up against a wall or lying over a folded blanket in a passive backbend, to restore your energy.

If you practice late in the evening, you may find that intense backbends or other postures that are stimulating to the nervous system prevent you from sleeping. Your emphasis should be on postures that are quieting and soothing.

Breathing. Remember to breathe through your nostrils at all times. Breathing through the mouth is tiring and puts additional strain on the heart.

Follow the instructions for breathing for each particular posture. As a general rule, movements that open the chest are done with a deep inhalation; movements that fold the body are done with a deep exhalation; and normal breathing is maintained while holding the posture. For

One cannot understand the rhythms and meanings of the outer world until one has mastered the dialects of the body.

TIMOTHY LEARY

example, when coming into Uttanasana (Standing Forward Bend) from Tadasana (Mountain Pose), you raise the arms overhead with a deep inhalation and bend forward from the hips with an exhalation. The breath remains quiet while you are in the posture. To come out of Uttanasana, you again extend the arms overhead with an inhalation to raise the torso, then bring your arms down to your sides with an exhalation.

Holding the posture. How long you hold a posture depends on your individual strength and stamina. If you feel exhausted after your practice session, you have been holding too long or working too hard. Try to adjust your pace so that you end your practice feeling rejuvenated. Pay attention to your inner clock.

In general, most postures may be held for half a minute to one minute. Once you are in the posture, turn your attention inward and focus on the lengthening of the spine or the quality of the breath. Keep your eyes open so that you remain alert and observant. When practicing a posture to the right and to the left, be sure to hold it for an equal amount of time on each side. After completing a posture, stand or sit quietly for a few breaths before beginning the next posture.

Resting postures may be held for five to ten minutes, or as long as feels beneficial. Allow your eyes to close gently and observe the movement of the breath as you begin to release deeper levels of tension and fatigue.

Pain. In our yoga practice, we must learn to distinguish between stretching sensations that are intense but beneficial, and pain that announces a potentially damaging maneuver. As a general rule, do not continue practicing a posture when you feel a sharp pain in or around the joints, in particular, the knees, hips, lower back, or neck. When you feel such a pain, first try to modify the posture by using a prop or support or by not coming into the posture so deeply. If the pain persists, eliminate this particular posture from your practice until you are able to consult with an experienced teacher. Pain usually means that you are not properly aligned in a posture and are stressing the joints. Trying to "work through" the pain can aggravate an existing injury. Learn to work with your body, not against it.

Menstruation. During the menstrual period, women should not practice inverted postures, such as Shirshasana (Headstand) or Sarvangasana (Shoulderstand). It is also advisable to avoid strenuous standing postures and intense backbends during this time. The most beneficial postures during menstruation include sitting forward bends, such as Janu Shirshasana (Head-to-Knee Pose) and Paschimottanasana (Sitting

Equanimity and peace in all conditions, in all parts of the being is the first foundation of the Yogic status. Peace is the first condition without which nothing else can be stable.

SRI AUROBINDO

51

Forward Bend), with the upper body supported on blankets or bolsters, or Suptabaddha Konasana (Supine Bound Angle Pose), with a bolster supporting the upper body, and Shavasana (Corpse Pose).

Pregnancy. During the first three months of pregnancy, all postures may be safely practiced with the exception of abdominal strengthening postures, such as Navasana (Boat Pose). During the second and third trimesters, continue to practice the standing postures to maintain your strength and stamina. Sitting forward bends should now be modified, so that you practice with the back concave and the front of the spine fully extended. All seated twists, with the exception of Bharadvajasana (Bharadvaja's Simple Twist), should be eliminated at this point, because they compress the abdomen. You may continue to practice inverted postures until you notice that your breathing becomes heavy. Finally, concentrate on postures that will help you with an easy delivery: Upavishtha Konasana (Open Angle Pose), Baddha Konasana (Bound Angle Pose), and Suptabaddha Konasana (Supine Bound Angle Pose). For Shavasana (Corpse Pose), try lying on your side with the top leg bent and your knee supported by a bolster.

Warming-up postures. Always begin your practice with two or three postures that help to warm the body and relieve initial stiffness. Warming up postures: Standing Leg Stretches, Adhomukha Shvanasana (Downward-facing Dog Pose), Adhomukha Vrikshasana (Handstand), and Surya Namaskara (Sun Salutation).

Standing postures. Standing postures develop the strength of the legs and the flexibility of the pelvis and lower back. They are important for learning basic principles of alignment and establishing a firm foundation. Tadasana (Mountain Pose) is the most fundamental standing posture. We move into other standing postures from Tadasana and return to it after completion. When coming out of a posture, return to Tadasana for two or three breaths before moving to the next posture.

If you feel at all fatigued after a standing posture, come into Uttanasana (Standing Forward Bend) or Prasarita Padottanasana (Widespread Forward Bend) as a resting posture. Students with very tight hamstrings and those with a history of lower back problems should practice Prasarita Padottanasana rather than Uttanasana, or bring the hands onto the wall for Wall Push.

Common standing postures are Tadasana (Mountain Pose), Vrikshasana (Tree Pose), Trikonasana (Triangle Pose), Uttanasana (Standing Forward Bend), Parshvakonasana (Side Angle Pose), Prasarita Podottanasana (Wide-spread Forward Bend), Virabhadrasana I & II (Warrior Pose I & II), Ardha Chandrasana (Half Moon Pose), Parshvottanasana (Intense Side Stretch Pose), and Parivritta Trikonasana (Revolved Triangle Pose).

As a general rule, practice the postures that are easier before the ones that are more difficult. For example, basic standing postures such as Trikonasana (Triangle Pose) will help you to warm up before you attempt the more advanced standing postures, such as Ardha Chandrasana (Half Moon Pose) or Parivritta Trikonasana (Revolved Triangle Pose).

Balancing postures like Vrikshasana (Tree Pose) and Ardha Chandrasana (Half Moon Pose) can be practiced against a wall if your balance is unsteady.

Inverted postures. Common inverted postures are Adhomukha Vrikshasana (Handstand), Adhomukha Shvanasana (Downward-facing Dog Pose), Shirshasana (Headstand), and Sarvangasana (Shoulderstand).

Sarvangasana (Shoulderstand) is one of the most important postures from a physiological point of view. By reversing the effects of gravity, the pressure on the abdominal organs is relieved, circulation to the upper chest is improved, and the thyroid gland in the throat is stimulated. Altogether, Sarvangasana has a very soothing and therapeutic effect. If practiced incorrectly, however, it can be damaging to the neck. Therefore, if you have had a neck injury or whiplash, you should consult with a qualified teacher before practicing this posture on your own.

Setu Bandhasana (Bridge Pose) is an excellent preparatory posture for Shoulderstand, helping to open the chest and shoulders and lengthening the neck without too much weightbearing. Beginners may use a chair to support the pelvis in Sarvangasana, or a wall to support the feet, before moving into the center of the room. As with Shirshasana (Headstand), described below, build your holding time very gradually over a course of several months or even years. Start with holding for a minute, and add an additional minute for each few weeks of practice. Eventually you will be able to hold Sarvangasana for ten minutes.

While in Sarvangasana you may practice the one-legged variations, Ekapada Sarvangasana (Shoulderstand with One Leg Extended Forward) and Parshvaikapada Sarvangasana (Shoulderstand with One Leg Extended to the Side), which stretch the hamstrings and release the hips. From Sarvangasana come into Halasana (Plough Pose) as a resting position and counterposture. Hold Halasana for about half the length of time that you held Sarvangasana. That is, if you hold Sarvangasana for six minutes, hold Halasana for three. Those with lower back problems or tight hamstrings may bring their feet onto a chair or wall for Halasana.

Prepare yourself for Shirshasana (Headstand) by practicing another posture that helps to open the shoulders, such as Adhomukha Vrikshasana (Handstand), Gomukhasana (Cow's Head Pose), or Adhomukha Shvanasana (Downward-facing Dog Pose). Immediately before Shirshasana, practice a posture in which the head is lower than the hips, such as Uttanasana (Standing Forward Bend) or Adhomukha Shvanasana, so that the blood does not rush suddenly to your head as you come up into Shirshasana. Likewise, when coming out of Shirshasana, rest for a few moments in Child's Pose with your head down, so that your circulation has a chance to adjust.

I recommend that you learn Shirshasana from an experienced teacher, especially if you have had any neck or shoulder problems. When you begin to practice Shirshasana on your own, hold for half a minute to one minute and build your time gradually over the course of many months. Practice near a wall if your balance is unsteady.

If you develop pain or acute discomfort in the neck during or after Shirshasana, discontinue practicing the posture until you have consulted with your teacher. If you practice Shirshasana, be sure to do Sarvangasana (Shoulderstand) later in the sequence. Shoulderstand is the counterposture for Shirshasana, as it lengthens the neck.

Backbends. Common backbends are Setu Bandhasana (Bridge Pose), Shalabhasana (Locust Pose), Dhanurasana (Bow Pose), Ushtrasana (Camel Pose), Urdhvamukha Shvanasana (Upward-facing Dog Pose) Urdhva Dhanurasana (Upward Bow Pose).

Backbends open the chest, stimulate the nervous system and increase vitality. When practicing backbends, we need to develop the strength of the legs and buttocks and the flexibility of the shoulders and upper back in order to protect the lower back from injury. Standing postures in general and Virbhadrasana I (Warrior Pose I) in particular help to prepare us for backbends. Handstand and other shoulder-opening postures are also good preparations. After backbends, do one or two twisting postures to relieve any discomfort in the lower back. If you experience acute pain during backbends, or feel discomfort afterward, consult your teacher.

Twisting postures. Common twisting postures are Bharadvajasana

(Bharadvaja's Simple Twist), Marichyasana I & III (Marichi's Seated Twist I & III).

Twisting postures help to neutralize the spine and give a gentle massage to the internal organs. However, if you move into a twist by gripping the diaphragm, you will restrict the breath and the posture will be exhausting. When practicing twisting postures, remember to lengthen the spine on the inhalation, and deepen the twist on the exhalation, keeping the diaphragm soft and wide.

Sitting postures. Common sitting postures are Dandasana (Staff Pose), Virasana (Hero Pose), Virasana II (Hero Pose II, also called Child's Pose), Gomukhasana (Cow's Head Pose), Janu Shirshasana (Head-to-Knee Pose), Tryanga Mukhaikapada Paschimottanasana (Seated Forward Bend with One Leg in Hero Pose), Paschimottanasana (Seated Forward Bend), Upavishtha Konasana (Open Angle Pose), Baddha Konasana (Bound Angle Pose).

Sitting forward bends are soothing for the nervous system and quieting for the mind. Initially, however, the tightness of the hamstrings make these postures very difficult. Sitting at the edge of a folded blanket will make them easier to execute. If you have lower back problems or are unable to take hold of the feet in seated forward bends, use a strap around the feet and keep the front of the spine fully lengthened. If you feel any discomfort after practicing seated forward bends, try one or two twisting postures or a supine posture such as Supta Padangushthasana to relieve your lower back, or simply lie on your back and bring your knees up to your chest.

Supine and resting postures. Common supine and resting postures are Supta Padangushthasana (Supine Head-to-Foot Pose), Supta Virasana (Supine Hero Pose), Suptabaddha Konasana (Supine Bound Angle Pose), Viparita Karani (Supported Shoulderstand), Shavasana (Corpse Pose).

Supine and resting postures may be practiced at the end of your routine to leave you feeling rejuvenated after your session. They may be practiced as a routine of their own when you are feeling especially fatigued or recovering from illness. When practicing them for therapeutic or restorative purposes, use a bolster to support the upper back and a blanket to support the head and neck. You may wrap a bandage lightly around your eyes, or place a cloth over your eyes to make it more soothing. These resting postures may be held for five to ten minutes each, or even longer.

Program One (forward bending sequence):

Standing Leg Stretches, Adhomukha Shvanasana (Downward-facing Dog Pose), Tadasana (Mountain Pose), Trikonasana (Triangle Pose), Uttanasana (Standing Forward Bend), Parshvakonasana (Side Angle Pose), Prasarita Padottanasana (Wide-spread Forward Bend), Ardha Chandrasana (Half Moon Pose), Parshvottanasana (Intense Side Stretch Pose), Adhomukha Shvanasana (Downward-facing Dog Pose), Shirshasana (Headstand), Sarvangasana (Shoulderstand), Halasana (Plough Pose), Dandasana (Staff Pose), Janu Shirshasana (Head-to-Knee Pose), Tryanga Mukhaikapada Paschimottanasana (Seated Forward Bend with One Leg in Hero Pose), Paschimottanasana (Seated Forward Bend), Upavishtha Konasana (Open Angle Pose), Baddha Konasana (Bound Angle Pose), Marichyasana I (Marichi's Seated Twist I), Shavasana (Corpse Pose).

Program Two (backbending sequence):

Adhomukha Shvanasana (Downward-facing Dog Pose), Adhomukha Vrikshasana (Handstand), Tadasana (Mountain Pose), Vrikshasana (Tree Pose), Trikonasana (Triangle Pose), Uttanasana (Standing Forward Bend), Parshvakonasana (Side Angle Pose), Prasarita Padottanasana (Wide-spread Forward Bend), Parivritta Trikonasana (Revolved Triangle Pose), Uttanasana (Standing Forward Bend), Adhomukha Shvanasana (Downward-facing Dog Pose), Urdhvamukha Shvanasana (Upward-facing Dog Pose), Shalabhasana (Locust Pose), Dhanurasana (Bow Pose), Ushtrasana (Camel Pose), Urdhva Dhanurasana (Upward Bow Pose), Bharadvajasana (Bharadvaja's Simple Twist), Marichyasana III (Marichi's Seated Twist III), Virasana II (Hero Pose II, or Child's Pose), Adhomukha Shvanasana (Downward-facing Dog Pose), Viparita Karani (Supported Shoulderstand), Shavasana (Corpse Pose).

Program Three (inverted posture sequence):

Surya Namaskara (Sun Salutation), Tadasana (Mountain Pose), Trikonasana (Triangle Pose), Uttanasana (Standing Forward Bend), Parshvakonasana (Side Angle Pose), Prasarita Padottanasana (Wide-spread Forward Bend), Virabhadrasana II (Warrior Pose II), Virabhadrasana I (Warrior Pose I), Uttanasana (Standing Forward Bend), Adhomukha Shvanasana (Downward-facing Dog Pose), Gomukhasana (Cow's Head Pose) in Virasana (Hero Pose), Supta Virasana (Supine Hero Pose), Shirshasana (Headstand), Setu Bandhasana (Bridge Pose), Sarvangasana (Shoulderstand), Ekapada Sarvangasana (Shoulderstand with One Leg Extended Forward), Parshvaikapada Sarvangasana (Shoulderstand with One Leg Extended to the Side), Halasana (Plough Pose), Supta Padangushthasana (Supine Hand-to-Foot Pose), Shavasana (Corpse Pose).

BALANCE IN YOGA
BY DONNA FARHI

Postures that require balance are unique in that they bring us up against our limitations and weaknesses in a very immediate way. How we respond to this self-confrontation is a surprisingly accurate indication of our internal state.

Balance is scary. It is a state of dynamic poise in which our usual sense of the body, together with our self-definition, seem to disappear. Usually we oscillate between extremes—in our lives as well as in our yoga practice. But when we maintain moderation, conflicts dissolve and we find ourselves in the pregnant fullness of the moment.

We are so used to living with conflict and difficulty that the difficulty becomes a comfort to us, because it is familiar. On some level we may even enjoy our pain, reveling in the histrionics of each crisis. If we can skillfully redirect our efforts to the task at hand, we can liberate a tremendous untapped resource of energy within ourselves.

When you are having trouble balancing in a posture, ask yourself these four questions:

1. What is the problem? (e.g., I am falling to the left)

2. What are possible causes of the problem?

3. What are some possible solutions to the problem?

4. What is the best solution at this moment?

Although this may sound absurdly simple, it is often the last approach we take. Too often, we approach difficulty in yoga by simply "trying harder." This strategy rarely works. Perhaps this is why balancing poses raise the ire of the more macho among us: Brute force will not do the trick. Only through skill does balance come.

To be "still" is divine, but we are humans, sometimes fragile and closed, sometimes strong and open. In our reach toward divinity, we have to fully embrace our humanity and be able to laugh at the falls and tumbles. In fact, I believe students are truly progressing in yoga when they can respond to ungraceful falls with laughter instead of curses.

Our cultural indoctrination has taught us to consider balancing as

Know ye not that your bodies are the members of Christ?

I CORINTHIANS 6:16

57

This body is mortal. It is subject to death. Yet it is the resting place of the immortal, incorporeal Self (atman).

CHANDOGYA UPANISHAD

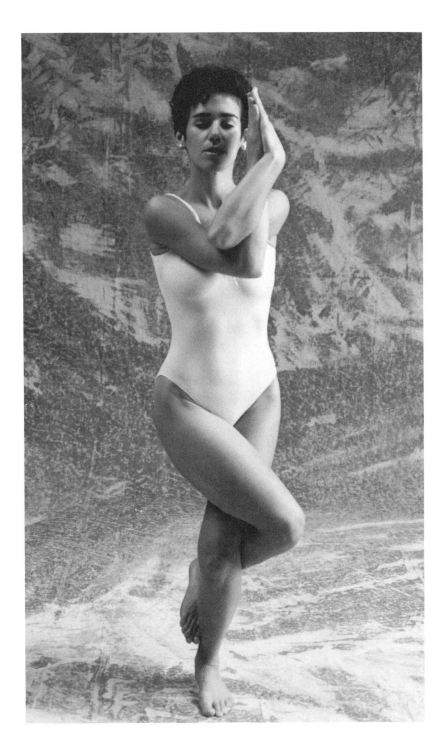

going beyond nature and "controlling" the body. In a sense, we approach balance as if it were an unnatural state. I believe that attitude began with the industrialization and mechanization of our world, when we switched from a respectful partnership with our environment to a relationship of domination whereby nature became something to be overpowered and bent to our will. All too often in our culture, "stillness" is translated in action as "rigidity" or "holding."

In the West we tend to see the body as separate from the psyche, representing an independent part of nature that must be curbed and kept subservient to our wishes. Whether conscious or unconscious, this is the paradigm we've inherited. And yet, in the fullest sense of the word, "to balance" can mean to *merge* and intersect with our environment and other people. Ultimately, our practice of yoga need no longer seem separate from the life processes around us.

One way in which a feeling of separation arises is through constricting or holding the breath, as often occurs when we attempt to balance. Although this "hold-on-whatever-the-cost" method may afford us the small ego gratification of "doing" the pose, it will never give our practice an organic sense of connection to the environment, nor the light, transparent quality that comes to the body when the breath moves freely, without constriction. To attain this freedom, we must rediscover the body's innate intelligence, connecting ourselves to the world in such a way that the postures are literally sculpted from the substance of the Earth.

The Origins of Balance: Human Crawling and Walking

As children mature and begin to crawl, they move first in what is known as a *homolateral* pattern, the type of movement in which the right arm and right leg move together, then the left arm and left leg. (This is the way camels move.) Later, the child learns to crawl in the *contralateral* pattern that will be the foundation for coordinated walking and sports activities later on.

Contralateral movement is the type of movement in which opposite arms and legs work together. This is the normal pattern in human walking and in most mammalian locomotion. Yet it is in the earlier homolateral pattern that we learn, or fail to learn, many of our balancing skills.

A clear example of how homolateral movement functions to keep us upright can be seen in the pedaling action of a unicyclist. When the right leg is pushed downward, the spine and ribcage move to the right

59

while the head remains centered over the tailbone and the cycle. If the cyclist were to flex toward the weight-bearing side, the bike would rock precariously to the right and overturn. This is a gross example of the more subtle and refined (and therefore more difficult to see) homolateral integration that takes place in walking.

People lacking development of the homolateral pattern tend to walk very quickly because they are literally falling forward in space. When they slow down, they are amazed to find that they can no longer balance.

Students who have difficulty balancing in the standing postures consistently lack ability in the homolateral pattern or are restricted from integrating the pattern into their movement because of muscular tightness. Students lacking ability in the homologous pattern of pushing and reaching also have difficulty balancing because they cannot sufficiently extend the body in order to stabilize the center of gravity over the base of support.

Vrikshasana (Tree Pose)

Stand in Tadasana (Mountain Pose) with the feet hip-width apart. As you shift your weight to the right foot, turn the left leg out and place the heel of the left foot gently on the inner ankle of the right foot. Taking hold of the ankle with the left hand, raise the left leg up and place the foot firmly on the inner right thigh. Check to be sure that you are not bending toward the right side. The torso should slightly extend over the weight-bearing side, and the hips should both be the same distance from the floor. If the left hip rises as you place the foot on the inner right thigh, you may be trying to outwardly rotate the left hip too much. To correct this problem, bring the left knee forward, lower the hip until it is even with the right side, and then work to bring the knee back *without raising the hip*. Use the support of a chair or wall, if necessary.

When your balance is firm, extend both arms strongly downward with the hands outstretched. The more you press the right foot into the floor and reach the arms downward, the easier it will be to lengthen the spine upward. Now bring the hands together in the namaste (prayer) position in front of the sternum. Expand the ribs with the breath in order to broaden the shoulders as you extend the elbows away from the body.

Breathe fully into the upper lungs until you feel the cavity of the chest expanding. On an inhalation, extend the arms over the head and interlock the thumbs. As you breathe up into the lungs, feel that the arms are propelled skyward like an arrow by the inspired breath. This will be counterbalanced by the strong movement of the pelvis and feet downward into the floor. A moment will come when this upward movement of the chest and breath will urge the head to look upward. When this happens, shift your focus to a point on the ceiling and balance for a few moments longer. Repeat on the other side.

Balancing Tips

Vision. In the beginning, focus on a spot at eye level in front of you. As you become more confident, open up your peripheral vision so that you become aware of yourself balancing in relationship to the environment around you. Notice that when you harden your eyes and focus on one spot, the muscles (especially the erector spinae muscles of the back) tighten and move toward the center of the body. When you open up your peripheral vision, the muscles "echo" the visual opening by expanding away from the center of the body.

Step by step (or, "You don't have to do it all at once"). Make the task of balancing easier by using the support of a wall or chair. When you feel confident, graduate to the next level of difficulty.

Concentration. The quality of your concentration is important. If your concentration is hard, like a vise gripping the body, balancing will be even more difficult. Let your concentration rest on the body like dust resting on the surface of a table. Like the quality of your vision, the body will echo the quality of your concentration.

Broaden your base of support. When in doubt, broaden your base of support, first by broadening the sole of the foot, then by widening your stance. In a pose such as Handstand, increasing the distance between the hands will make balancing easier.

Feet. The feet will be your foundation for most of the balancing postures. Your feet may be compressed and twisted from years of wearing fashionable shoes or walking incorrectly. Work carefully in all the standing poses to broaden and lengthen the feet, especially by extending the toes. If you have weak arches and ankles, be especially aware of lifting the arch of the foot in all poses, while simultaneously pressing the base of the big toe. You may want to consider having some deep tissue massage or seeing a good podiatrist if stiffness or pain is a consistent problem.

Where does the body end and the mind begin? Where does the mind end and the spirit begin? They cannot be divided as they are interrelated and but different aspects of the same all-pervading divine consciousness.

B. K. S. IYENGAR

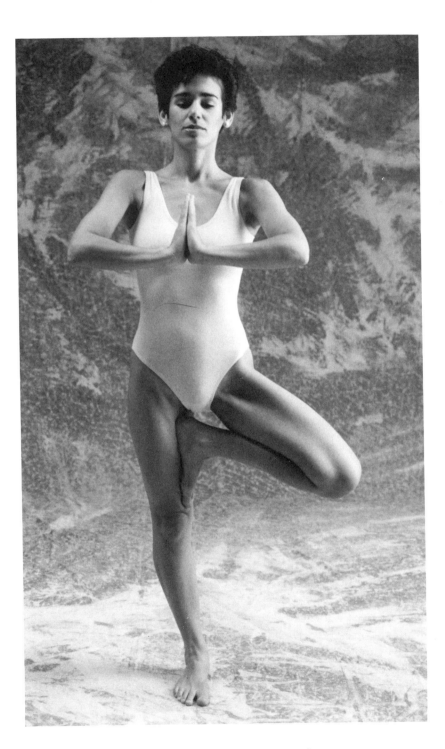

Breathing. Holding the breath and hardening the diaphragm are common strategies used to create steadiness in balancing poses. This kind of balance is precarious at best, and the body will appear to be contracting inward toward the center. Tightening the diaphragm is a normal reaction when the weight is too far back on the heels or when the spine is hyperextended, so check for these more obvious errors. More often, though, holding the breath is a habitual response to difficulty that has become deeply encoded in the nervous system and will take patience and time to correct.

Just before you attempt any balancing pose, check that your breathing is calm and regular and that the area around the front lower ribs is pliant. Like a surfer riding a wave, let the full length of the exhalation carry you into the movement. Continue to breathe fully throughout the duration of the posture. As you inhale, bring your awareness to your center. As you exhale, remain in touch with this center as you let your awareness expand, just as a full-blown dandelion flower expands in all directions but is held together in the center. When you begin to extend your awareness further and further out away from the center of the body, the balance of the pose will derive less and less from the skeleton and muscles and more and more from the force moving through the spaces between the joints. The body will feel tremendously strong and delightfully transparent when it is aligned in this way. By breathing and expanding our awareness fully in this way, we bring all that is external to us literally inside ourselves, thereby merging with all that is.

You must savor the fragrance of a posture.

B. K. S. IYENGAR

HOW TO GROW A LOTUS: LEARNING THE LOTUS POSTURE
BY DONNA FARHI

If you are one of the many millions of Westerners who find the Lotus Pose difficult, take heart! Now you can ease your way into *Padmasana*.

Throughout childhood, and especially in the typical adult sedentary job, prolonged sitting on chairs has caused a shortening of the very muscles and ligaments that need to be flexible for Padmasana. To make matters worse, the hip is an extremely deep ball-and-socket joint with some of the strongest ligaments in the body, which prevent the femur from becoming dislocated. With this stability comes a subsequent lack of mobility. To change the structure of the hip takes careful, persistent practice over a long period of time.

Never force yourself into Padmasana or the other cross-legged poses. The knee joint is particularly susceptible to injury for a number of reasons. First, the knee is one of the most primitive joints in the body and is much weaker than the hip. If you have very tight hips, you may overstretch the knees without increasing your hip flexibility one iota. The hips, not the knees, must be flexible for the Lotus Pose.

Second, when fully extended, the knee joint will not rotate. When the joint is bent, however, a slight rotation does come into play, and this rotation can be injurious to the knee, damaging ligaments, cartilage, and meniscus. The knee is an unforgiving joint; once injured, it may never be the same again. Therefore, if you feel a sharp pain in the knee, adjust your position or seek the help of a competent teacher.

The following series will help you prepare for Padmasana. The stretches are best done after practicing standing poses when the body is warmed up. Those who are tight should practice in the afternoon, when they have more flexibility. Begin by holding each position one minute, increasing to five minutes as the poses come with more ease. Use a watch or timer for consistency, as one minute can rapidly become 15 seconds in the more intense stretches.

Those with knee or ankle injuries should be especially cautious here. If your discomfort cannot be alleviated by adjusting your position, you would be wise to seek the help of an experienced teacher. You might also try alternative sitting positions, such as the Hero Pose (Virasana) or the Sage Pose (Siddhasana) with the buttocks elevated on a firm blanket. These poses are excellent for both meditation and breath control.

In all the stretches, use deep abdominal breathing to open the body from the inside. Rather than "trying" to relax by pressing the muscles into the stretch, take your breath deep into the center of the pelvis. With each inhalation feel the hips expand, and with each exhalation allow the muscles to slip away from the bones. Working gently in this way, the body will welcome the pose and progress quickly toward the achievement of Padmasana.

Lunge One

This pose stretches the ligaments and muscles of the external rotators of the bent leg and the psoas and groin of the straight leg.

Sit with the heel of the right foot in line with the pubic bone. Extending the other leg straight behind you, with the kneecap facing downward, sink the right hip into the floor. Keep the chest lifted to take the weight of the pelvis off the femur. Repeat on the other side.

Not only the flower of the lotus, but the posture itself, appears so glamorous that its achievement seems worthwhile, regardless of its difficulty. It is called the "royal posture" and one who can do Padmasana with ease is fortunate. It is as if one assumes, with the lotus posture, the beauty, the grace, and the divinity of the flower.

SWAMI SIVANANDA RADHA

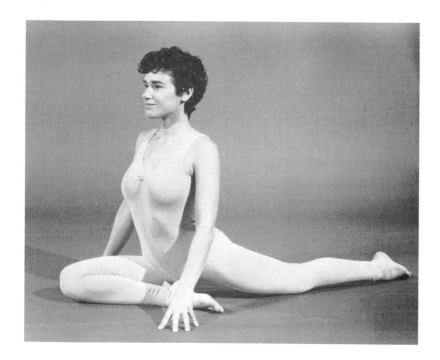

LUNGE ONE

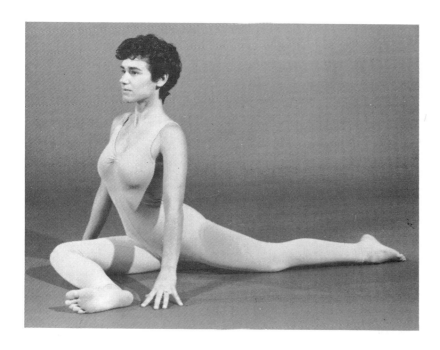

LUNGE TWO

Lunge Two

To make the lunge stretch more intense, move the foot away from the thigh until the upper and lower legs form a right angle. Keeping the knee on the floor to stabilize the joint, attempt to move the left hip toward the floor.

Reclining Hero Pose (Supta Virasana)

This pose lengthens the psoas and quadriceps muscles of the thigh, especially above the knee.

Sit in Virasana (Hero Pose) with the knees in line with the hips. Drawing the center of the pelvis into the center of the thighs, recline back onto the elbows. Depending on your flexibility, either support the back with a bolster or recline on the floor with the arms over the head. Do not attempt to recline if the knees splay out or come off the floor.

Through-the-Hole Stretch

This pose stretches the external rotators.

Lie on your back with both knees bent. Cross the left leg so that the outside of the calf is resting on the right thigh. Take the left arm through the gap of the left leg around the back of the right thigh. Clasp hands. As you draw the right thigh toward you turn the left hip out and move the left knee away from you to open the hip. Repeat on the other side.

Seated Angle Pose (Upavishtha Konasana II)

This pose stretches the hamstrings, adductors, and groin and the lateral hip and buttock area.

Sit with the legs spread wide apart. Turn the torso to face over the right thigh. Elongate and twist the spine as you bend over the extended leg. Press the opposite hip down to increase the stretch on the lateral side of that hip and buttock.

Bound Angle Pose (Baddha Konasana), variation

This pose stretches the adductors and lateral hip.

Sit in Baddha Konasana with the hands clasped around your feet. Hold one minute. Now elevate the feet in front of you on a book or folded blanket. Use the arms to keep the spine in an upright position, moving the torso toward the feet. Hold for up to five minutes. Now try Baddha Konasana with the feet on the floor. You may be surprised at how much closer the knees are to the floor.

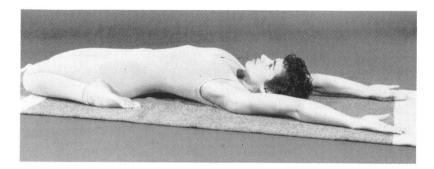

RECLINING HERO POSE
(*Supta Virasana*)

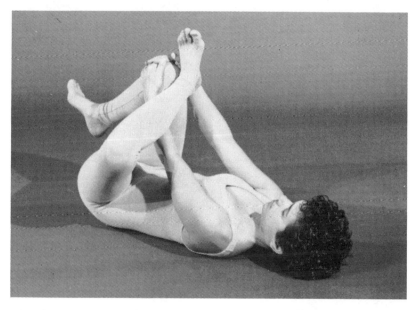

THROUGH-THE-HOLE
STRETCH

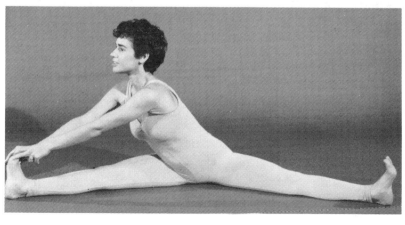

SEATED ANGLE POSE
(*Upavishtha Konasana II*)

BOUND ANGLE POSE
(Baddha Konasa), variation

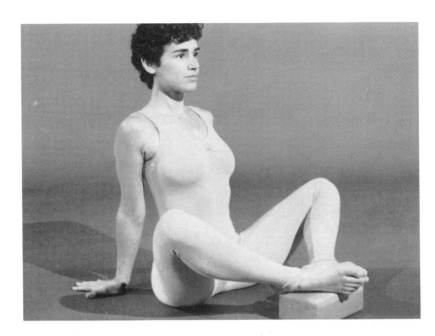

COW FACE POSE
(Gomukhasana)

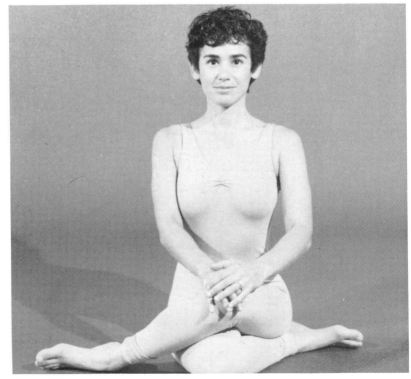

Cow Face Pose (Gomukhasana)

This pose increases elasticity in the hips, legs, and ankles.

Sit with the legs extended straight in front of you (i.e., in the Staff Pose, or Dandasana). Raising your seat, bend the right knee back and sit on the right foot. If this is too difficult, place a folded blanket between the buttock and the heel. Now cross the left leg over the right so that the knees are resting on top of one another and the left foot is turned under. Place the hands on the thigh and press the knees firmly together. Repeat, changing the cross of the legs.

Reclining Leg Stretch (Supta Padangushthasana), variation

This pose stretches the lateral rotators and psoas of the extended leg.

Lie flat on the back with the legs extended straight. Bend the left knee and taking hold of the feet in both hands, draw the knee down and out toward the floor next to the right rib cage. Press the right thigh down as much as possible.

Head-to-Knee Pose (Janu Shirshasana)

This pose stretches the lateral rotators, hamstrings, and adductors.

Sit in the Staff Pose (Dandasana). Bend the left knee and draw the leg up and out to the side. Rotate the left thigh out as much as possible. Turn the torso to face toward the big toe of the extended leg, and pivot forward from the hips into a forward bend over the right leg.

Tailor's Stretch

This pose stretches the lateral rotators.

Sit in a simple cross-legged position. Now move the feet away from the groin until both legs form right angles. Maintaining this position, tip forward with a straight spine until you feel a deep stretch in the outside of the hip. Repeat, changing the cross of the legs.

Cradle Stretch

This pose stretches the lateral rotators and adductors.

Sit in the Staff Pose (Dandasana). Bend the left knee and turn the leg out. Place the sole of the foot in the crease of the right elbow and the thigh in the crease of the left elbow. Clasp hands. Gently move the hip back and forth, rotating the hip outward as you do so. To increase the intensity of the stretch, keep moving the left foot away from the floor until the leg forms a right angle. Go on to the next posture before practicing the Cradle Stretch on the right.

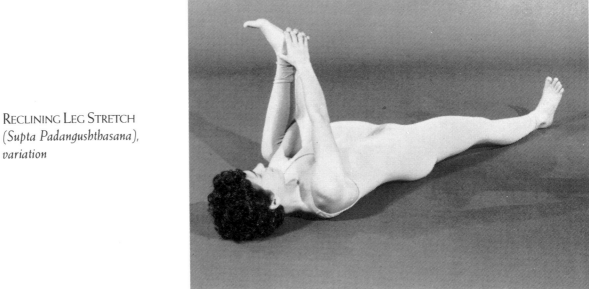

RECLINING LEG STRETCH
(*Supta Padangushthasana*),
variation

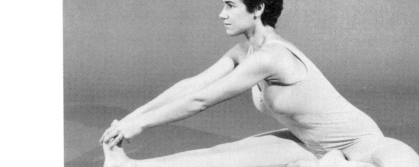

HEAD-TO-KNEE POSE
(*Janu Shirshasana*)

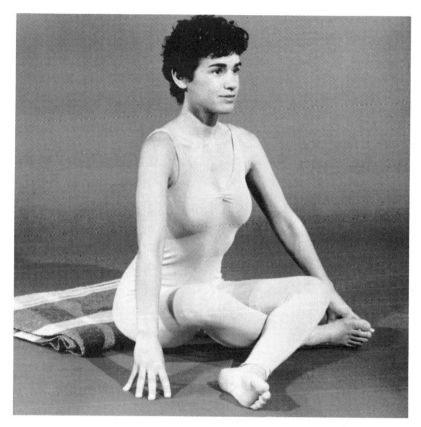

TAILOR'S STRETCH

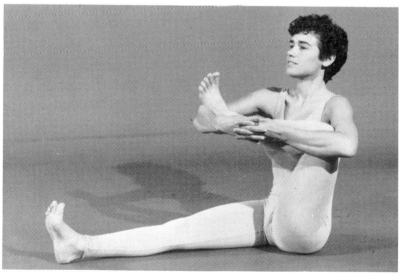

CRADLE STRETCH

Seated Forward Bend in the Half Lotus Pose
(Ardhabaddhapadma Pashchimottanasana)

From the Cradle Stretch, place the ankle on top of the right thigh so that the heel is pressing into the lower abdomen. If you are unable to bring the heel to the abdomen, place the ankle farther down the thigh. Support the knee with a folded blanket if it does not reach the floor. By supporting the knee in this way, you make it possible for the muscles of the hip to gradually let go. Toward the end of your stay in the pose, remove the prop—you may be surprised to find that the knee moves with ease toward the floor.

When bringing the foot onto the top of the thigh for Padmasana, hold at the shin and ankle, not at the top of the foot. Keep the ankle flexed to prevent supination, or "sickling." Once the ankle is resting on the thigh, you may relax the foot. "Sickling" can pull on the ligaments and cartilage of the lateral knee, causing potential injury to these delicate structures.

Sage Pose (Siddhasana)

Siddhasana is relatively easy to practice and provides an excellent warm-up for Padmasana. It can also be used as an alternative to Padmasana in meditation. Bring the right heel in line with the pubic bone. Place the left ankle on top of the right, with the toes of the left foot between the thigh and calf of the right leg. Sit with the weight on the sitting bones (ischial tuberosities). If the lower back rounds, elevate the buttocks with the folded corner of a blanket. Sit for five minutes. Now change the cross of the legs.

Lotus Pose (Padmasana)

Sit in the Staff Pose (Dandasana), using a firmly folded mat to elevate the hips. Keeping the spine erect, bring the right leg into the Cradle Stretch position. Extend the inside of the right ankle as you externally rotate the right hip. With the foot flexed to prevent rotation at the knee and ankle joints, place the right foot on top of the left thigh.

The sole of the foot should be pointing to the side, rather than up at the ceiling, and should press gently into the lower abdomen. Once the ankle is resting on the thigh, you may relax it. Now bend the left knee and cross the leg in front of you. Grasp the lower shin of the left leg and gently lift up into the right thigh to complete the pose. The left knee will be slightly above the floor. If necessary, support it with a folded blanket.

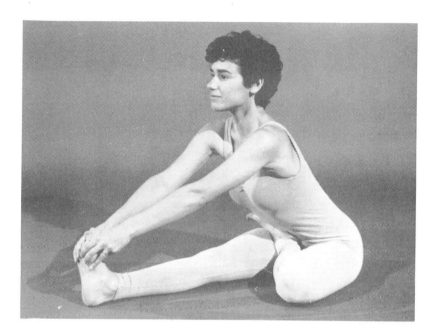

SEATED FORWARD BEND IN
THE HALF LOTUS POSE
(*Ardhabaddhapadma
Pashchimottanasana*)

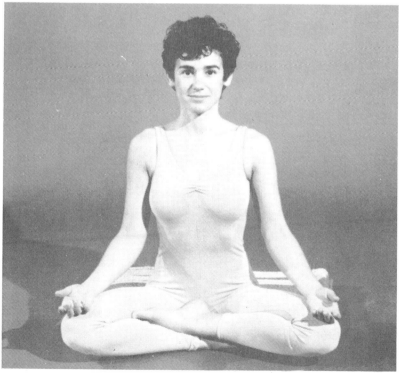

SAGE POSE
(*Siddhasana*)

LOTUS POSE
(*Padmasana*)

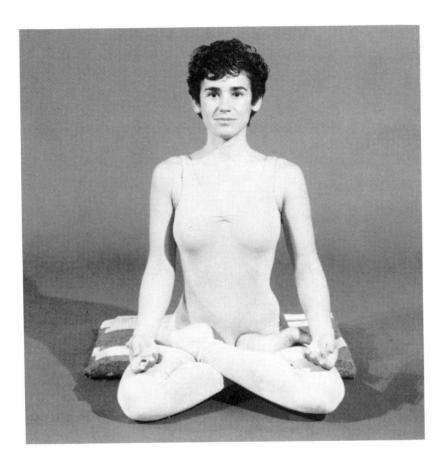

Sit with the center of the diaphragm balanced over the center of the pelvis so that the breathing is free. Maintaining the lift and breadth of the sternum and chest, rest the hands on the knees with the palms facing up. Begin by staying in the pose for brief periods, increasing your stay as your hips become more flexible. Change the cross of the legs and practice on the other side.

Do not despair if you cannot lift the second leg up into the full position. Continue with the preparatory stretches and try practicing the Half Lotus Pose (one leg in Full Lotus, the other crossed tailor-style underneath). Gradually increase the length of stay in the Half Lotus as you feel the hips becoming more flexible. Like Siddhasana, the Half Lotus may be used as a meditation posture in its own right. Just be sure to alternate legs from session to session to correct the imbalance inherent in the pose.

In practicing Padmasana, remember that the body and the asana must meet on their own terms in their own time. If you inflict the asana on the body, you may set up a dichotomous relationship between what you think the body "should" be and what the body is. The body then becomes an enemy to be conquered rather than a companion on the journey. By giving up your preconceived ideas and images of how far you think you should go, you free yourself to explore the asana in the present moment, just as a lover might give full attention to his beloved. Practicing with true affection, let the pose become a journey rather than a destination. Then even a difficult pose like Padmasana will become enjoyable.

RESOURCES

Books

Cunningham, Annalisa. *Stretch and Surrender*. Cambridge, MA: Rudra, 1992.

Couch, Jean. *The Runner's Yoga Book*. Berkeley, CA: Rodmell Press, 1990.

Mehta, Silva, et al. *Yoga: The Iyengar Way*. New York: Knopf, 1990.

Scaravalli, Vanda. *Awakening the Spine*. San Francisco: HarperSanFrancisco, 1991.

Tobias, Maxine, and John Patrick Sullivan. *Complete Stretching*. New York: Knopf, 1992.

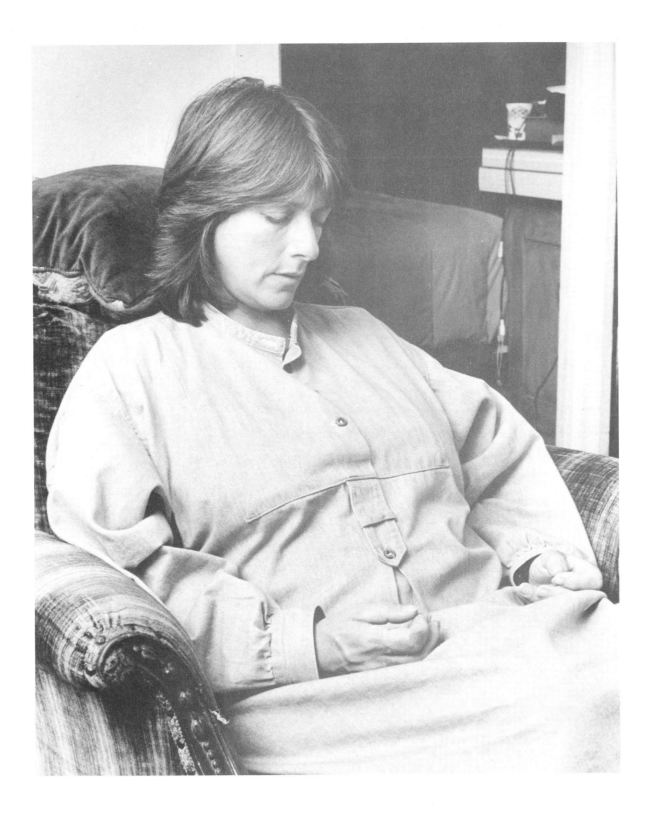

FOUR

Yoga for Health

Yogis recognized long ago that in order to accomplish the highest goal of yoga, which is the realization of the Self, or God consciousness, a healthy physical body is essential. For when we are sick, our attention is seldom free enough to contemplate the larger Reality, or to muster the energy for yogic practice. The masters of yoga also teach us that personal growth is possible only when we fully accept our embodiment and when we truly understand that the body is not merely skin and bones but a finely balanced system of energies. Yoga can help us catch up with the great discovery of quantum physics: $E = mc^2$. Another way of putting this mathematical truth is: mind over matter.

Although yoga is best used as preventive medicine, some of its practices also have great therapeutic value. They can help those suffering from various difficult physical conditions, like back pain, scoliosis, and arthritis. This chapter contains several essays specifically dealing with such conditions, and it also includes articles on how to improve immune system responses and overcome menstrual problems. These offer a lot of encouragement to sufferers. However, ideally, your yoga practice should be an integral part of your efforts to maintain good health and prevent degenerative diseases.

Yoga is not a religion, it is crystallized truth.

SELVARAJAN YESUDIAN
AND ELISABETH HAICH

INTRODUCTION TO THERAPEUTIC YOGA

The word "therapy" comes from the Greek verb *therapeuein,* meaning "to heal, to take care of." Yoga can be understood as a comprehensive approach to healing, for it goes to the root of all disease, which is our false relationship to life itself. We fall ill when our body-mind is out of balance, when the life force fails to circulate freely in us. Ultimately, there can be no complete healing until we have restored our primal trust in life, which alone removes all those obstructions within us that tend to manifest as ill health.

Most of our diseases are symptoms of an underlying dis-ease: our sense of being cut off from the sustaining power of life. We feel separate, isolated, alienated, ill at ease. As we become aware of this feeling, which we share with billions of others, we experience the need for wholeness. We begin to understand that we are not *really* sealed off from life but are in fact interconnected with everything and everyone else. At times, this intellectual understanding may be confirmed and enriched by an actual experience of unity and wholeness. Now we are well on the road to balance, harmony, healing, and well-being. Not every illness is a sign of our loss of primal trust. Nevertheless, it is always an opportunity to strengthen that trust and to grow emotionally and spiritually.

Yoga seeks to foster that condition of wholeness in which, even if we should experience a spell of misfortune and illness, we nevertheless feel restored to life and healed in our relationship to the larger Reality. Yoga is radical spiritual therapy.

For millennia, yoga has had a close connection with *Ayurveda*, which is India's traditional medical and healing system. According to Ayurveda, which literally means "science of life," body and mind form an interactive system. This is also the viewpoint of yoga. Both schools of thought also insist that a healthy, wholesome life must be happy and morally sound. Moreover, the authorities of Ayurveda and yoga both recommend the cultivation of self-knowledge and serenity, which ensure our well-being.

Western medicine is slowly rediscovering these ancient fundamental insights about disease, health, and wholeness. But we do not have to wait for our family doctor to catch up with avant-garde physicians like Bernie Siegel, Elisabeth Kübler-Ross, Larry Dossey, Deepak Chopra, Andrew Weil, and other prominent doctors in the field of alternative and holistic medicine. We can assume responsibility for our own healing and at the very least inform ourselves.

There is a growing literature on Ayurveda, traditional Chinese medicine, homeopathy, herbalism, aromatherapy, color therapy, bodywork, healing touch, and so on. Magazines like *Yoga Journal* and *Natural Health* (the former *East West Journal*) contain much useful information

Illness contains an inner code by which it wants to "say something."

LARRY DOSSEY

about new books and current activities, such as lectures and workshops. More than ever, we do not need to be passive victims of our illness or the medical system.

RESOURCES

Books

Carlson, R., and B. Shield, eds. *Healers on Healing*. Los Angeles: J. P. Tarcher, 1989.

Frawley, D. *Ayurvedic Healing: A Comprehensive Guide*. Salt Lake City: Passage Press, 1989. A significant work, trying to make Ayurveda accessible to the Western health-conscious reader.

Frawley, D., and V. Lad. *The Yoga of Herbs*. Santa Fe: Lotus Press, 1986.

Gerber, R. *Vibrational Medicine*. Santa Fe: Bear & Co., 1988. A pioneering work which takes the Einsteinian model of the universe as energy seriously.

Heimlich, J. *What Your Doctor Won't Tell You*. New York: HarperCollins, 1990.

Inglis, B. *Natural Medicine*. London: Fontana, 1980.

Justice, B. *Who Gets Sick: How Beliefs, Moods, and Thoughts Affect Your Health*. Los Angeles: J. P. Tarcher, 1987.

Klein, A. *The Healing Power of Humor*. Los Angeles: J. P. Tarcher, 1989.

Liberman, J. *Light: Medicine of the Future*. Santa Fe: Bear & Co., 1991. An exploration of the many therapeutic uses of light.

Melville, A., and C. Johnson. *Health Without Drugs*. New York: Fireside Books, 1990.

Olsen, K. G. *The Encyclopedia of Alternative Health Care*. New York: Pocket Books, 1989.

Periodicals

Natural Health. This is a bimonthly magazine packed with information about healthcare and obtainable at most newsstands. The offices are located at 17 Station Street, Brookline Village, MA 02147-1200

Yoga Journal. For information and address, see the resources for Chapter 1.

Organizations

American Holistic Medical Association, 2727 Fairview Avenue E, Seattle, WA 98102. Tel. (206) 322-6842. The association makes available a list of physicians practicing holistic medicine in the United States. It also has a booklet entitled *How to Choose a Holistic Health Practitioner.*

American Institute of Vedic Studies, P.O. Box 8357, Santa Fe, NM 87504. The institute is directed by David Frawley, who offers a comprehensive correspondence course in Ayurveda.

Lotus Light, P.O. Box 2, Wilmot, WI 53192. Tel. (414) 862-2395. A good source for herbs and herbal products, including Ayurvedic products.

World Research Foundation, 15300 Ventura Boulevard, Sherman Oaks, CA 91403. Tel. (818) 907-5483. The Foundation provides information about the Healing Research Center, which is in the process of being created as an alternative medicine/healing center, based on the principles of energy medicine formulated by Richard Gerber, M.D.

BOOSTING THE IMMUNE SYSTEM
BY MARY PULLIG SCHATZ, M.D.

Your Body Hears What You Say

The body responds to its own conscious and unconscious communications, and a variety of signals are interpreted as stress—e.g., tight jaw; tense muscles in the abdomen, upper back, and neck; poor posture; mental agitation. Status reports are constantly being sent through language, coping behavior, breathing patterns, posture, and health practices. If these reports indicate danger or threat, resources are shifted toward the stress response, with its negative effects on immunity. On the other hand, messages of safety and well-being encourage a shift toward the relaxation response, creating an environment that enhances immune function.

Coping Behavior

How one reacts to stress has more influence on immunity than the severity of the actual stressful event.[1] A number of studies have corre-

There is no such thing as my body, or your body, except in words. Of the one huge mass of matter, one point is called a moon, another a sun, another a man, another the earth, another a plant, another a mineral.

SWAMI VIVEKANANDA

lated positive coping behavior with healthy immune function, and poor coping behavior with defective immune function.

Of the personality traits associated with low resistance to disease, feelings of helplessness are especially destructive to immunity in times of stress.[2] Just knowing that there is something constructive to be done is protective of immune function. Even if the actual situation cannot be changed, reducing stress levels through relaxation and breathing techniques has been shown to mitigate negative effects on immunity.[3,4]

Another way to look at coping involves the concept of "locus of control." Studies have shown that people with an external locus of control believe that events are entirely unrelated to their choices and decisions, and that they are helplessly adrift in a chaotic world. This chronically stressful environment depresses immunity. Conversely, people with an internal locus of control believe that, through active participation, they can exert a definite influence on events in their life. Rather than as calamities, events are experienced as natural developments based on conscious choices. As feelings of helplessness decrease, the stress response lessens and the immune system flourishes.[5]

Health Practices

Positive and negative health practices speak directly to the body and, through it, to the immune system (see chart on page 84). Enjoyable exercises,[6] yoga postures, and restorative relaxation[7] reinforce the message that all is well, and that normal immune function is appropriate. Every instance of choosing, preparing, and eating healthful and nourishing food, in amounts commensurate with one's needs, is received as good news.[8] The body thinks, "I must be worthy of life; I am being so well-fed, well-exercised, and well-rested. Let me be well."

When one continues negative health practices such as smoking and ignores the resultant danger signals (cough, chronic bronchitis, etc.), the body gets a message of low self-esteem, and its defenses are lowered. This stressful, psychologically depressed state, combined with repetitive tissue injury from inhaled smoke, leads to diseases of immune failure such as cancer.[9]

Body Language

Body language is read by the nervous system and translated as a signal either of danger or of well-being. According to studies, facial expressions alone can cause changes in the involuntary nervous system.[10]

Whether stress does us in depends largely on how we view our troubles and what chemical messages we trigger in our brains.

BLAIR JUSTICE

Consider how the body might respond to the position of depression—bowed head, slumped chest, furrowed brow.

By now, readers who are also students of yoga have probably recognized that so many "recently discovered" psychological and physiological determinants of good health are indeed integral components of the ancient science and philosophy of ashtanga yoga, the eightfold path of Patanjali. There is a clear correlation between yoga and the positive health practices documented in the medical literature. And this list will certainly grow as Western medicine further explores the mind-body relationship.

Circulation

A regular, balanced, and varied practice of classical asanas is an ideal exercise program to keep the immune system healthy. The many salutary effects of yoga postures and breathing on circulation are well-documented. Good circulation is crucial to all phases of the immune reaction. Immune cells travel through the bloodstream and lymphatic fluid to patrol the body for invaders. Since not every helper T cell can recognize every invader, it is necessary to assist helper T cells in getting around to all their checkpoints. Exercising the "muscle pump," "chest pump," and "heart pump" with each asana helps immune surveillance by promoting the circulation of macrophages and helper T cells. Improving circulation promotes two-way communication between immune cells and the hypothalamus, the pituitary, lymphoid tissues, and other target organs.

Yoga postures that squeeze, soak, and spread (create space in) the organs of immune surveillance (skin, gastrointestinal tract, respiratory tract) also promote strong defenses at these important body frontiers.

Conscious Breathing

The body constantly monitors the quality (rate and depth) of the breath as well as its effectiveness (blood concentrations of oxygen and carbon dioxide). Shallow, agitated respirations are read as "Danger: Initiate stress response!" Breathing with paced respirations (as in pranayama or the stress-reducing breathing technique of B. K. S. Iyengar) reduces arousal and anxiety in threatening situations.[11]

The conscious breathing system of pranayama provides a direct avenue of communication to the self.[12] The practice of pranayama quickly induces the relaxation response and its accompanying enhancement of immunity. The improved blood oxygenation associated with

A balanced and optimistic attitude, healthy lifestyle habits in regard to diet, and basic care of the human body will support the optimal function of not only our immune system but our entire body.

ELSON M. HAAS

more complete chest expansion is another message of good news to the inner self. Continuing to return the attention to the breath teaches that one need not respond to every arising thought. This is a practical lesson in developing an internal locus of control. As events in the mind can be influenced through conscious choice, so can events in life. Aside from the formal practice of pranayama, simple breathing techniques can be practiced anytime, anywhere, to rapidly reduce tension and anxiety.

Sympathetic/Parasympathetic Balance

According to B. K. S. Iyengar, the practice of asana and pranayama "balances the nadis (you call them nerves) and the sympathetic and parasympathetic nervous systems."[13] These two divisions of the automatically functioning portions of the nervous system govern internal organs and blood vessels (e.g., heart rate, blood pressure, unconscious breathing, digestion). A predominance of sympathetic impulses creates the stress response, with its readiness for fight or flight. Predominance of the parasympathetic components creates the relaxation response, which restores energy and heals the body.

The relaxation response experienced during the Corpse Pose (Shavasana), meditation, pranayama, and the restorative poses promotes healthy immune surveillance and responsiveness. In particular, the restorative poses offer a way to benefit from the relaxation response in a supported position that conserves and restores energy, while enhancing circulation and respiration.

Communication to the Self

Think of the yogic asana as mime—the architecture of each pose communicates not with others, but with the inner self. With the language of the asanas, one counteracts the feelings of helplessness and weakness so destructive to immunity. Each asana strengthens one's internal locus of control. The body becomes an actor, not a reactor. Self-worth is enhanced.

The vigorous standing poses exhibit strength and confidence and reinforce those personality characteristics, furthering internal locus of control. The backbends teach that flexibility, openheartedness, and strength can coexist. The forward bends demonstrate physically an environment safe enough from danger that vigilance can cease. The inversions and arm balances teach balance and poise in difficult and/or disorienting situations. One learns that when the mind is centered and the breathing quiet, energy can be directed into constructive solutions,

The phenomena of focused attention, imagery, biofeedback, and therapeutic hypnosis all operate by altering the direction of blood flow. Altering blood flow by directed thinking, imagining, and feeling is one of the basic, common factors in the resolution of most, if not all, mind-body problems.

ERNEST LAWRENCE ROSSI

One must live as if one had ten thousand years. Only out of this leisure will real richness and intensity be born. This Leisure is at the centre of the universe.

LEWIS THOMPSON

83

rather than wasted in the free-floating anxiety and helplessness so harmful to immune defenses. Self-imposed limitations relax as tight muscles lengthen and body carriage improves.

The postures and pranayama provide the opportunity to explore the self and observe how it reacts to life's challenges and surprises. One's yoga practice can be a personal growth laboratory for working out in body and mind what can soon be applied to daily life. With time, one realizes that one can control how one responds to events, just as one can control how one responds to an intense stretch of the hamstrings or the fear of one's first full arm balance.

Yoga provides the means to become physically fit in the context of a philosophy that encourages positive health practices and personality characteristics. The body is no longer divorced from the mind and the spirit. Rather, the body is the vehicle for growth and spiritual development—and the immune system becomes the guardian of high-level wellness.

HEALTH PRACTICES, ATTITUDES, AND IMMUNITY

Enhances Immune Function	Depresses Immune Function
Health Practices	
Good nutrition	Poor diet (poor quality, improper quantity)
Proper exercise	Inactivity
Adequate sleep	Insomnia, somnolence
Relaxation, meditation	Constant stress
Breathing practice or paced respiration	Smoking
	Heavy alcohol consumption
Approach to Life	
Active approach to illness	Resigned, helpless approach to illness
Optimistic, positive outlook	Pessimism
Change seen as opportunity for growth	Change seen as threat
Internal locus of control	External locus of control
Inner stability, equanimity	Agitation, emotional volatility
Appropriate self-confidence	Too much or too little self-confidence
Sense of purpose, commitment	Apathy
Social support system	Isolation
Involvement	Alienation
Warm relationship with others	Poor communication with others

Relief from Back Pain
by Mary Pullig Schatz, M.D.

If you've ever suffered from an aching back, you know that the pain always seems to strike at exactly the wrong time—when you're doing your holiday shopping, for example, or racing to meet an important business deadline, or boarding the plane for a long-overdue vacation, or taking care of a sick child.

Yoga stretches and relaxation techniques can be powerful tools for coping with stress-induced back pain. Although yoga can't make a stressful situation go away, it can change the way you perceive and respond to it.

Being in danger or feeling helpless causes a specific set of physiological responses designed to prepare you to fight or flee. The fight-or-flight response is characterized by increased heart rate, blood pressure, mental alertness, and muscle tension. A chronically stressed state can keep your body's healing mechanisms from working, prolonging recovery from injury or disease and leading to stress-related diseases, including ulcers, alcoholism, high blood pressure, depression, and, of course, back pain.

Stress also exaggerates postural strain by increasing muscle tension. This increase in muscle tension does not occur uniformly throughout the body. Muscles that are already irritated, tense, or injured are more vulnerable. Any musculoskeletal misalignment is exaggerated, increasing the likelihood of reinjury.

Gentle yoga stretches and relaxation techniques help break this self-perpetuating stress cycle. The brain perceives muscle stretch as the opposite of muscle tension. Whereas a muscle in spasm sends signals of danger to the entire body, the message of yoga muscle stretches is one of safety and well-being.

Resting Your Back

Therapeutic, constructive rest is important in back rehabilitation. You may usually think of a resting position as being reclining or semireclining, but these positions can harm a recovering back. Lounge chairs and soft sofas are frequent culprits. An example of destructive rest is the couch-potato syndrome—lying with the spine rounded for hours, munching on snacks. In such situations, back pain can result from prolonged inactivity, poor posture, and weight gain.

In contrast, resting in restorative yoga poses provides the following:

Conscious living trains the mind by relying on its natural propensity to create habits. . . . By practicing healthy attitudes and behaviors, even when our minds, unconvinced of their value, continue to be drawn to the momentary pleasure of unhealthy ones, we will slowly and permanently establish new, healthier, and more pleasurable habits.

Elliot S. Dacher

- Support of the body in a position of good alignment, in which tired, overworked muscles can completely relax.

- Gentle, passive stretch for tight or overworked muscles.

- Correction of some asymmetries in muscle length and tension.

- Elimination of accumulated mental or emotional stresses and tensions.

The relaxation poses described in this article are a good way to start doing yoga. Practice one or more of them every day. It is a good idea to do one or two resting poses before bedtime. These poses can also help you get the kinks out after a long trip or after mild trauma.

It's especially useful to practice relaxation poses before commencing an activity that's likely to challenge your back. The postures can help you begin the potentially dangerous activity with a better alignment, so injury is less likely to occur. They can remind your muscles and bones of good alignment principles, so you're more likely to use proper body mechanics as you pass through the danger zone. Afterward, they can help you return to correct alignment.

To practice relaxation poses, choose a place where you'll be neither too warm nor too cold. Lying on a folded quilt or blanket on the floor (rather than on a bed) is best. Be sure to use good body mechanics while getting down onto the floor and coming back up.

Make sure that you won't be disturbed. You won't be able to relax fully if you know that you may have to pop up to answer the phone at any moment. If you don't have an answering machine, take the phone off the hook. Let the world wait. If the room is cool or you tend to become chilled, dress warmly and have a blanket nearby.

Yoga Poses to Rest Your Back

Please note: The information contained in this article isn't intended as a substitute for medical treatment. Do not begin practicing these exercises until you have obtained a thorough evaluation of your condition and advice about the exercises from a qualified healthcare professional who is familiar with them. Consult your healthcare advisor:

- If you experience a worsening in severity or duration of pain after beginning this program;

- If pain persists even when you're lying down in one of the relaxation poses;

- If headache, vomiting, or fever develop in association with back pain;

- If back pain is associated with loss of bladder or bowel control;

- If one or both legs or arms develop weakness or numbness.

Elbows on the Table

Props needed: chair, table.

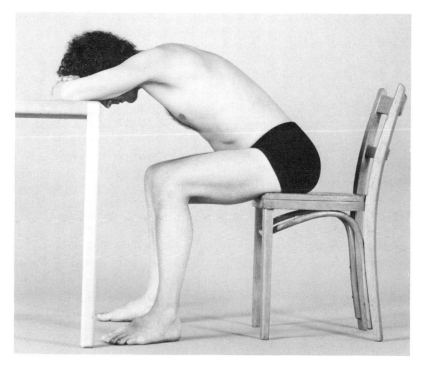

FIGURE ONE

Position and Adjustment

Sit in a straight chair on a nonslip surface in front of a table, so that you can comfortably lean forward onto the table. Rest your head and folded arms on the table (Figure 1). Avoid letting your lower back overarch. Soften your front lower ribs back into your body to slightly flatten the lumbar curve and stretch the paraspinal muscles (the muscles on either side of the spine). Hold this position for 20 to 30 seconds, breathing normally. Release and repeat several times, alternating the crossed position of the arms. (If you begin with the left forearm on top, place the right forearm on top the next time, and so on.) Always return to the erect sitting position slowly, breathing deeply, to avoid dizziness.

Breathing and Imagery
With each breath, allow your lower back to lengthen and release. Use the Relaxation Breath, breathing normally and pausing at the end of each exhalation for several seconds.

Rationale
This supported position allows the spinal muscles to release and lengthen so that the vertebrae can separate and allow the discs to expand. Resting the forehead in this way encourages the relaxation response by relieving the neck and shoulder muscles of their burden.

Notes

- If you have a flat lumbar curve, allow your lower back to arch slightly toward a more normal curve.

- This pose isn't suitable for those with spondylolysis or spondylolisthesis.

- This is a great back rester for those in late pregnancy.

Chair-Seated Forward Bend with Torso Support
Props needed: two chairs, four to six blankets. (As needed: thick towel.)

Position and Adjustment
Fold each blanket in half lengthwise, then fanfold it to create a rectangular support twelve inches wide. Stack the blankets neatly and place them across the seat of one of the chairs so that the long side of the stack is parallel with the back of the chair. (If you have yoga bolsters, they can be used instead.)

Sit in the other chair facing the side of the first chair. Separate your knees and pull the blanketed chair between your legs so that you're looking out over the long axis of the folded pile of blankets. Stretch your torso up as tall as is comfortably possible. Using your arms for support, lower your torso onto the pile of blankets (Figure 2). If possible, allow your forehead to rest on the blankets or turn your head to one side and rest there for several minutes. If your head doesn't reach the blankets, fold the towel and place it under your head. Increase or decrease the thickness of the chest support by adding or taking away blankets until you're comfortable. Allow your abdominal muscles to become soft and passive. Release your back with each exhalation.

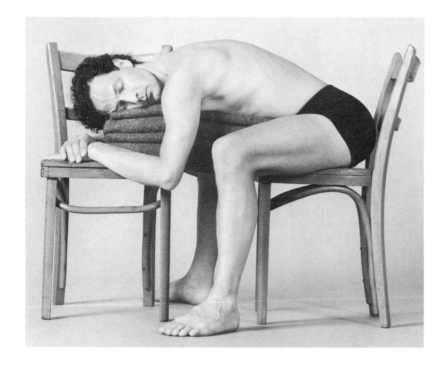

FIGURE TWO

To come up, use the support of your arms to push your torso back up to a seated position, keeping your abdominal and paraspinal muscles relaxed. (It's very important to use your arms, not your paraspinal muscles, to lift out of the pose—otherwise your paraspinal muscles might go into spasm.) Move quietly to the next pose.

Breathing and Imagery
Inhale and exhale normally. Pause briefly at the end of each exhalation to allow further spontaneous release of the breath. Allow your abdomen to gently expand with each inhalation. See the muscles of your back relaxing and releasing tightness and spasm. See your spine elongating. See pain and fatigue escaping the body with every exhalation.

Rationale
With the abdomen relaxed and the torso supported, the back muscles can relax and lengthen, allowing more space between the vertebrae for better disc nourishment and healing.

Note

- This pose isn't suitable for those with spondylolysis or spondylolisthesis.
- Don't practice this pose during the second half of pregnancy.

Child's Pose
Props needed: pad. (As needed: two twisted socks, rolled towel, folded blanket.)

FIGURE THREE

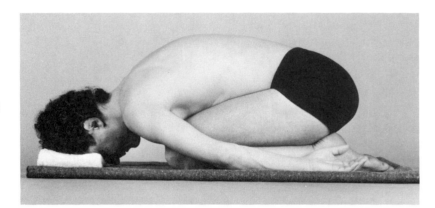

FIGURE FOUR

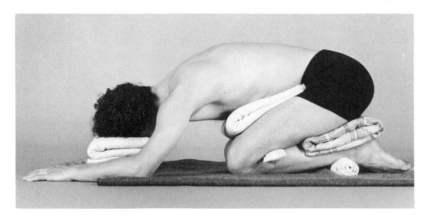

Position and Adjustment
Kneel and rest your chest on your thighs. Place your forehead on the floor or turn your head to one side. For comfort you can place a pad under your knees or your head or both (Figure 3). If you can't get your head on the floor, use a folded blanket of the proper height for head support. If your knees hurt, you can place a twisted sock in the bend of each knee to create more space. A rolled towel under your ankles can

relieve excessive stretch there. If your buttocks don't rest on your heels, place a folded blanket on your lower legs and sit on that (Figure 4).

Breathing and Imagery

Inhale into your abdomen and back. On each exhalation, release your spine and visualize it getting longer. As you go through several breath cycles, your trunk will actually passively elongate. To accommodate this elongation, lift your chest and abdomen off your thighs slightly, accept the new length, and rest again on your thighs. Stay here as long as you can, up to several minutes. Keep relaxing and lengthening into the pose. Sit up slowly, using the arms to support the trunk. Move quietly to the next pose.

Rationale

This is a relaxing, passive stretch for the muscles on either side of the spine. It teaches conscious relaxation of these muscles, which can stay tense without your being aware of it, and helps reeducate them to have a longer resting length. This allows more space between the vertebrae for the discs and decreases disc degeneration caused by constant compression.

Notes

- It's important to use the strength of your arms to push up to a sitting position. Otherwise your newly relaxed paraspinal muscles might go into painful spasm.

- If this posture bothers your knees, do Chair-Seated Forward Bend with Torso Support instead.

- This isn't a recommended position for those with spondylolysis or spondylolisthesis. If you have spondylolysis or spondylolisthesis, this and other forward bends can actually aggravate the tendency for forward slippage of the damaged vertebra.

- This pose can be practiced in the first half of pregnancy if the knees are separated widely to accommodate the growing baby and the belly isn't compressed against the floor. During the second half of pregnancy, practice this pose only as long as you can do so without compressing the abdomen.

From *Back Care Basics*, by Mary Pullig Schatz, M.D. Reprinted with permission of Rodmell Press, Berkeley, Calif. Copyright © 1992 by Mary Pullig Schatz, M.D.

YOGA AND THE MENSTRUAL CYCLE
BY JANE MACMULLEN

Yoga and PMS

Menstruation belongs to a cyclically ordered system. This blood mystery hints at a cosmos where life and death are as intertwined as are the fibers in spun yarn or the two snakes on the Caduceus.

GENIA PAULI HADDON

The menstrual cycle is created by fluctuations in the female sex hormones, which trigger signaling among the hypothalamus, pituitary, and ovaries.

Symptoms experienced during the pregestation phase of the monthly cycle are activated largely by the hormone progesterone in the luteal phase. This hormone causes the uterus to become engorged with blood, the breasts to become swollen and tender, and the kidneys to retain water.

Fluid retention in the tissues is what causes most menstrual discomfort; it arises mainly the day or two before menses begins. Therefore, premenstrual yoga asana practice would focus on relieving the pressure of fluid buildup. When the menses begins, the body naturally relieves itself of some excess fluid through more frequent urination and looser bowel movements. To further relieve fluid retention, we need to enhance venous and lymphatic drainage, which is the movement of blood and lymph back to the thoracic cavity, toward the heart. Improving venous drainage improves overall circulation and decreases the risk of varicose veins.

The lymphatic system is a "drainage" system consisting of vessels close to the capillaries of the cardiovascular system as well as lymph nodes, which play a vital role in the immune system. Lymphatic circulation drains approximately two to four liters from the tissues daily.

Once the blood moves into a capillary, most of the initial pressure imparted to it by the heart is lost; thus, other means are needed to move it through the veins back to the heart. Since the lymphatic system has no pump, similar mechanisms are needed to move lymph to the heart. Following is a list of five basic mechanisms that aid both venous drainage and lymphatic circulation. Included in each listing are suggested asanas to facilitate the mechanism. The asanas can be practiced before and during menses, but in the latter case you may choose to practice in a modified, supported, or passive manner. Long, fluid breathing is suggested throughout.

1. Gravity. Yoga is particularly helpful in moving fluid from the legs by elevating the lower body above the heart. Full inverted postures are excellent in this regard. If you are not practicing inversions, invert the legs up the wall. Practice other asanas that raise the legs.

2. Skeletal Muscle Action. The squeezing, milking action of skeletal muscles around the vessels by contraction and relaxation aids the movement of lymph toward the heart, where it can flow freely. A practice of repetitive movement rather than holding provides the desired action. The Sun Salutation (Surya Namaskara) is excellent for contraction and relaxation movements as well as for flowing breath.

3. External Pressure and Manipulation. Massage with a pressure/release action on the veins (like squeezing a sponge), as well as massage that includes lifting, rotating, twisting, or inverting limbs, will aid drainage. Massage can also be relaxing, nurturing, and emotionally supportive. Pressing one part of the body against another (distal to proximal; e.g., feet to groin, fingers to armpit) is another way to gain this effect. There are many asanas that accomplish this movement.

4. Respiration. Deep breathing or pranayama practice also facilitates venous and lymphatic drainage, as its suctionlike force pulls fluid from veins. In addition, it has a relaxing effect.

5. Smooth Muscle Action. Contracted fibers around the large veins near the heart are activated by excitement, which in turn enhances venous return. We can assist this process by working with the first four mechanisms.

Menstrual Cramps

Cramps may come from the effect of prostaglandins, hormonelike substances developed in the tissues that act locally (rather than traveling in the bloodstream). Prostaglandins play a role in the spasming of the spinal arteries, which leads to the sealing off of blood-engorged arteries but also causes menstrual cramps. (Incidentally, migraine headaches are also believed to be caused by spasming of the arteries due to prostaglandins.) Moderate cramps are a natural part of the process. When aspirin or premenstrual pain relievers are taken to ease cramps or headaches, they also interfere with the necessary sealing-off process.

Forward bends tend to press and release the lower abdomen, relieving cramping and lower back pain caused by referred pain from the uterus.

Lower back pain can also be relieved by standing postures, twists, forward bends, and massage. Backbends can ease the feeling of congestion in the front of the body and can also relieve lower back pain by extending and arching the spine (modified or supported as one chooses).

Regarding inversions: The anatomical design of the uterus does not promote backward flow of blood into the uterus. There is no evidence

Menstruation is not a painful process when we allow the natural period of time to have its own way with us. Yet by repressing the energies of the menstrual period, we find ourselves trapped in the lack of expression such repression manifests in our lives. . . . We must break the menstrual taboo.

VICKI NOBLE

that inversions cause endometriosis or increased uterine infection. During the menses there is a scenario in the uterus similar to the first month of pregnancy. We need to examine whether to practice inversions at these times, but up-to-date information is not presently available.

The Golden Womb

Although modern women lack the celebration of the lunar cycle that women in many traditional societies enjoy, we can tap into our own heightened intuition during menses and create rituals to nurture and embrace the divinity of our inner selves. The Golden Womb (Hiranyagarbha) is described in the ancient Vedas, the oldest scriptures of Hinduism, as the source of divine wisdom. When one is freed of the ego, the Vedas say, "the knowledge of the Golden Womb flows into one effortlessly and naturally." The contemporary yoga teacher Usharbudh Arya comments: "As a fetus receives nourishment from the mother through the umbilical cord, so all minds in meditation receive knowledge from the Golden Womb, the Teaching Spirit of the Universe."[14]

Menstruation is completely neutral: there is nothing impure about it. It all depends on the individual woman, on her thoughts and feelings and how she uses them.

OMRAAM MIKHAEL AIVANHOV

We are alienated, removed from our sources of power, and so we have developed menstrual cramps and premenstrual syndromes.

ZSUZSANNA E. BUDAPEST

RESOURCES

Books

Iyengar, G. S. *Yoga: A Gem for Women.* Palo Alto: Timeless Books, 1990.

Lark, S. *PMS Self-Help Book.* Berkeley: Celestial Arts, 1984.

Phelan, N., and M. Volin. *Yoga for Women.* London: Arrow Books, 1979.

Notes

[1] S. E. Locke et al., "Life Change Stress, Psychiatric Symptoms, and Natural Killer Cell Activity," *Psychosomatic Medicine*, no. 46 (1984), p. 441.

[2] M. L. Laudenslager et al., "Coping and Immunosuppression," *Science*, no. 221 (1983), p. 568.

[3] R. Glaser and J. Kiecolt-Glaser, "Relatively Mild Stress Depresses Cellular Immunity in Healthy Adults," *Behavioral and Brain Sciences*, no. 8 (1985), p. 401.

[4] S. O. Kobasa et al., "Hardiness and Health: A Prospective Study," *Journal of Personality and Social Psychology*, no. 42 (1982), p. 168.

[5]J. H. Johnson and I. G. Sarason, "Life Stress, Depression, and Anxiety: Internal-External Locus of Control as a Moderator Variable," *Journal of Psychosomatic Research*, no. 22 (1978), p. 205.

[6]H. B. Simon, "The Immunology of Exercise," *Journal of the American Medical Association*, no. 252 (1984), p. 2735.

[7]Glaser and Kiecolt-Glaser, *loc. cit.*

[8]M. C. Gershwin et al., *Nutrition and Immunity* (Orlando, FL: Academic Press, 1985).

[9]P. Hersey et al., "Effects of Cigarette Smoking on the Immune System," *Medical Journal of Australia*, vol. 2, no. 9 (1983), p. 425.

[10]P. Ekman et al., "Facial Expressions of Emotion and Involuntary Nervous System Changes," *Science*, no. 221 (1983), p. 1208.

[11]K. D. McCaul et al., "Effects of Paced Respirations and Expectations on Physiologic and Psychologic Responses to Threat," *Journal of Personality and Social Psychology*, no. 37 (1979), p. 564.

[12]B. K. S. Iyengar, *Light on Pranayama* (New York: Crossroad Publishing, 1981).

[13]_____, personal communication, Pune, India: February 1987.

[14]U. Arya, *Yoga-Sutras of Patanjali with the Exposition of Vyasa: A Translation and Commentary. Vol. 1: Samadhi-Pada* (Honesdale, PA: Himalayan International Institute, 1986), p. 69.

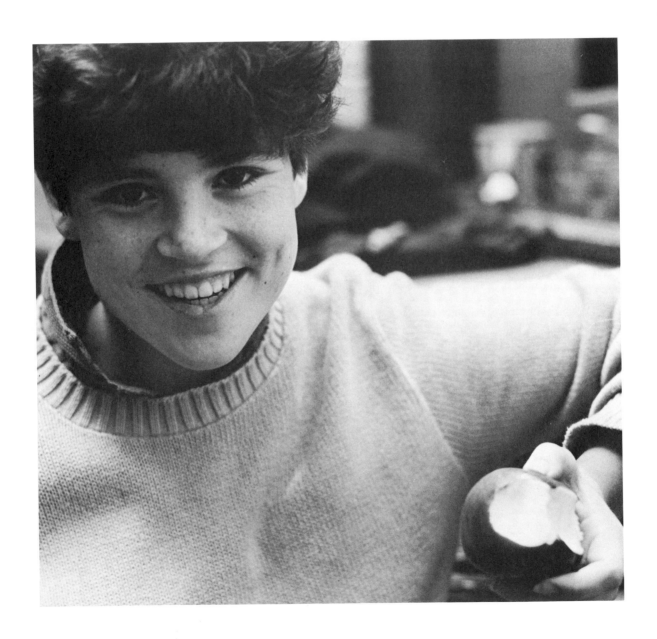

FIVE

Eating the Yoga Way

There is a growing recognition among healthcare practitioners that one of the most basic ways of ensuring our physical well-being is proper diet. This understanding amounts to a rediscovery of ancient knowledge, for the yogis of India have long emphasized the importance of eating right. This chapter will give you the fundamental principles of the yoga of food (anna yoga) and encourage you to inspect what and how you eat. Yoga is all-inclusive, and no aspect of human existence is ignored.

Tomorrow we will begin [studying the] Mandukya Upanishad. You can't understand Mandukya if you eat two meals a day—so now you'll have only one meal a day, at noon.

Swami Chinmayananda

TRADITIONAL PRINCIPLES OF DIETING

Thousands of years before modern psychosomatic medicine and therapy, yogis understood that body and mind are a functional unit, that mental states are mirrored in the body and vice versa. They were great experimenters, using their own bodies as their laboratories. By trial and error, as well as by virtue of their trained intuition, they learned a great deal about the impact of food on the body-mind—knowledge that is only now being slowly rediscovered.

They found that what we eat truly affects our inner life. One type of food promotes life, increasing our vitality, strength, health, and emotional buoyancy. A second type makes us agitated and causes pain and illness, while a third type makes us sluggish and ultimately leads to sickness.

These three nutritional categories traditionally have been regarded as manifestations of the three primary constituents of nature, which are called *sattva, rajas,* and *tamas* in Sanskrit. According to yoga philosophy, the interplay of these three forces is responsible for the entire web of creation. They have been compared to the principles of light, motion, and gravity respectively. However, they are not merely physical forces but also underlie all psychological processes. Thus sattva is the principle that is mentally and spiritually illuminating and uplifting, whereas rajas maintains the mind in constant tension and conflict. The third principle, tamas, is the most binding, for it causes us to be creatures of habit rather than innovative and spontaneous.

The food we eat reinforces our particular personality type, which can be predominantly sattvic (as in the case of yogis), rajasic (as in the case of most overactive Westerners), or tamasic (as in the case of "lazy" individuals). The yogic ideal is to cultivate the sattva factor in all matters, so that the mind becomes lucid, alert, and capable of higher spiritual realization.

Diet is a very important aspect of the yogic path to increasing purity, luminosity, serenity, and joy. It matters greatly what we eat, as well as how much and when. A favorite saying among contemporary yoga masters is: "You are what you eat." We can easily test this maxim in our own life. Simply observe the effect different foods and quantities of food have on your inner life.

The *Bhagavad Gita* (XVII. 8ff.), the most famous yoga scripture, contains these verses:

> Foods that promote life, lucidity, strength, health, happiness, and satisfaction, and that are savory, rich in oil, firm, and heart-gladdening are agreeable to the sattva-natured person.

> Foods that are pungent, sour, salty, spicy, sharp, harsh, and burning are coveted by the rajas-natured person.

> And that which is spoiled, tasteless, putrid, stale, left over, and unclean is food agreeable to the tamas-natured person.

The *Hatha Yoga Pradipika* (I.62), an important yogic manual from the medieval period, recommends a variety of grains, honey, milk, ghee, butter, several Indian vegetables, and pure water as promoting the sattva aspect. Modern dieticians would question some of these food categories. However, it must be remembered that some of the processes of hatha yoga, notably breath retention, greatly enhance one's metabolism. Indeed, advanced hatha yoga practice, involving the awakening of the body's psychospiritual energy known as the *kundalini,* particularly calls for a diet rich in fat. Clearly, we must neither offhandedly dismiss the

A mind consciously unclean cannot be cleansed by fasting.

MOHANDAS K.
("MAHATMA") GANDHI

98

dietary wisdom of yoga nor blindly follow it, but discover our own optimal diet. For some people, it will be a diet consisting predominantly of fruit and fruit juice, whereas others may require a more substantial diet.

While the yoga scriptures contain all manner of good advice about suitable foods, their single most important recommendation is to eat minimally and to fast periodically. Most of us in the West overeat, and yet, because of the poor quality of the processed foods we consume, many of us are overweight while at the same time being undernourished.

According to some yoga schools, disciplined eating is one of the basic moral observances (yama). The yogis and yoginis take care of their diet because they do not wish to do violence to the environment, both external and internal. They know that food can uplift as well as pollute them. Only a mind that is like a polished mirror can serve the hoped-for spiritual awakening. Therefore, we must take full responsibility for our dietary needs.

The most important dietary rule for longevity is systematic undereating.

DAN MILLMAN

RESOURCES

Books

Calbom, C., and M. Keane. *Juicing for Life.* Garden City, NY: Avery Publishing, 1992. An excellent guide to fresh fruit and vegetable juicing.

Cousens, G. *Spiritual Nutrition and the Rainbow Diet.* Boulder, CO: Cassandra Press, 1986. An intriguing treatment of the connection between diet and spiritual life.

Haas, E. M. *Staying Healthy with Nutrition.* Berkeley, CA: Celestial Arts, 1992. A tome of nearly 1200 pages containing much valuable information and a good bibliography for further exploration.

Kordich, J. *The Juiceman's Power of Juicing.* New York: William Morrow, 1992. A revolutionary program for staying healthy with juices by the well-known "Juiceman."

Robbins, J. *Diet for a New America.* Walpole, NH: Stillpoint Publishing, 1987. Essential reading for anyone interested in conscious living and eating.

———. *May All Be Fed: Diet for a New World.* New York: Morrow, 1992.

Schaeffer, S. L. *Instinctive Nutrition.* Berkeley, CA: Celestial Arts, 1987. The first English book on "anopsotherapy," making a strong argument for finding one's own appropriate diet by recovering the body's instinctive knowledge.

Organizations

Instinctive Nutrition Center, 6 Hurndale Avenue, Toronto, Ontario M4K 1R5, Canada. The center serves as a clearing house for instinctive nutrition.
The Juiceman (Jay Kordich), 655 South Orcas, Suite 220, Seattle, WA 98108.

All life is sacred, all life is one; no one has a right to question the sacredness of another, no one has a right to commit violence against another.

SHREE PUROHIT SWAMI

NONHARMING (AHIMSA) AND THE VEGAN DIET
BY VICTORIA MORAN

"Don't change your diet," my first yoga teacher had told me. "Yoga will change your diet." And it did. Within months, I had replaced meat and stimulants like coffee with gentler fare from nature. As I learned more about the yogic concept of reverence for all life, the notion of "total" or "pure" vegetarianism became more and more appealing. Pure vegetarians, or *vegans* (vee-guns), live completely on products from the plant kingdom, eschewing not only meat and fish but eggs and dairy products as well. They thereby divorce themselves from all exploitation of the so-called "food animals" who comprise 95 percent of the animals killed by human beings every year.

The traditional yogic diet has through the centuries been lacto-vegetarian. Eggs have largely been avoided due to their rajasic or stimulating quality. Also, because they contain the potential for a sentient creature to develop, yogis have advised against their use in keeping with the ideal of ahimsa, non-killing, or, more generously translated, "doing no harm." Yogic literature has ascribed to milk and its products the sattvic character. That is, dairy foods are said to be readily digested, easy on the system, and thus conducive to spiritual practices. Taking them does not directly kill an animal, and the respect given cows in India is widely known, albeit often misunderstood.

On grounds of ahimsa, however, many yoga students and other people today have come to realize that dairy foods provided by modern agricultural methods are not as innocent as they appear. With only 3 percent of the American population farming for the rest of us, "intensive" or "factory" systems of agriculture are the norm. This means that male calves are often separated from their mothers at birth so that the milk provided by nature for the young animal can instead be taken for human use. The calf is either slaughtered immediately ("bob veal") or sent to the wretched confines of a tiny, bare stall where he is fed an anemia-producing diet and allowed no exercise.

These practices enable him to render the gourmet's prize of "white veal" at the end of his short life. Many concerned people, even non-vegetarians, do not eat this veal. Vegans would remind them, however, that it is their demand for milk that spawned the veal industry. And dairy cows themselves, tireless "wet nurses to humanity," end their lives at the slaughterhouse.

Intensive systems for keeping laying hens in absurdly overcrowded conditions in small crates stacked one upon the other further fuel the argument of vegans and vegetarians who choose not to use eggs. But what about eggs from the kindly family farmer down the road whose chickens are out pecking in the dirt like chickens are supposed to do? And what's wrong with taking milk from the neighbor's goat or cow after she has nursed her youngster? To these certainly reasonable queries, most vegans would return another question: Why? They would remind us that nearly every hen will end up in the soup pot eventually, and besides, eggs with their notorious cholesterol and fat content are certainly not necessary items of diet. Milk, too, was certainly meant to feed the young of that species. Only the human, say vegans, is never weaned, and this "baby food" is not good for us.

Simply for reasons of health, then, many people have adopted totally vegetarian eating habits. Cardiologists have long seen its benefits: as early as 1961, even the conservative *Journal of the American Medical Association* editorialized that a completely vegetarian regimen "could prevent 90 percent of our thrombo-embolic disease and 97 percent of our coronary occlusions." Recent literature in the scientific community continues to support this statement and to point to a plant-based diet, low in fat and rich in complex carbohydrates, as the food plan of choice in the prevention and treatment of certain cancers, diverticular disease, diabetes and hypoglycemia, gall bladder problems, gout, obesity, and numerous other medical conditions. This easy, money-saving style of eating has also been shown to be ideal for pregnant and lactating women, growing children, and athletes. *The McDougall Program*, a 1990 book by John A. McDougall, M.D., and Mary A. McDougall, sifts the clinical and research findings into "human language" for a most convincing presentation of the physical benefits of a vegan diet.

Such a life-style, if widely undertaken, could also potentially benefit the health of our planet and the starving and malnourished people with whom we share it. How a vegetarian diet theoretically frees up vast quantities of grain for human consumption, rather than filtering it into economically inefficient flesh foods, was first presented to most of

We are to live so that no harm or pain is caused by our thoughts, words or deeds to any other being. In a positive sense, this means that we must cultivate love for all, and try to see the one Atman within everybody.

SWAMI PRABHAVANANDA
AND CHRISTOPHER
ISHERWOOD

If there is any single cause for which I would go up and down the land on a twentieth-century crusade, it is that of the meatless diet.

PAUL BRUNTON

us in Frances Moore Lappe's best-selling *Diet for a Small Planet*. A diet using no animal products is the most efficient of all in terms of land use and maximum yields per acre. Also, veganism makes tremendous sense environmentally. It uses far less land, water, and fossil fuel than a meat diet.

But is a vegan diet safe? Is it difficult? Is it boring? Varied meals of fresh, unrefined foods from the plant kingdom can provide ample nutrition. The only component necessary for human health not supplied dependably in a totally vegetarian diet is vitamin B12. For this, vegans are encouraged to get the minuscule amount of B12 required through regular use of fortified nutritional yeast or a vitamin supplement. In addition, many common cereals, such as Nutri-Grain and Kellogg's Bran Flakes, are fortified with B12.

As for protein, "It's impossible *not* to get enough protein on a vegan diet, provided you're eating natural foods," says H. Jay Dinshah, president of the American Vegan Society. Those "natural foods" that make up vegan fare are vegetables (including legumes), fruits, whole grains, nuts, and seeds. Bean/grain combinations and soy foods like tofu provide large amounts of protein, and even leafy greens are surprisingly rich in this nutrient. Kale, mustard greens, spinach, and broccoli, as well as almonds, tofu, and sesame seeds, are also abundant sources of calcium. (Much less calcium is required by vegetarians than by meat-eaters, and among traditional groups who use no animal foods, osteoporosis is unknown—even among women who bear and breastfeed an average of 10 children.)

When preparing meals at home, you can be a vegan gourmet, and cookbooks can become intriguing resources. Eating out can be a fascinating excursion to a natural foods or ethnic restaurant, or you can order a simple salad and baked potato meal just about anywhere. And veganism carried beyond diet can bring ahimsa into play in many areas of life. Finding alternatives to cosmetics and household cleaners that contain animal ingredients or have been tested on living animals is a challenge many vegans accept. They also look for clothing of non-animal fabrics and healing systems not dependent on drugs (which are usually tested on animals).

The resultant life-style is an individual adventure. Veganism is much like yoga in that you learn about it, it strikes a chord and then becomes your own. And with veganism, as with yoga, subtle changes come about: You suddenly realize you are a little slimmer, a little happier, a little more at peace.

Resources

Books

Braunstein, M. *Radical Vegetariansim: A Dialectic of Diet and Ethic.* Los Angeles: Panjandrum Books, 1981.

McDougall, J., and M. McDougall. *The McDougall Plan.* Piscataway, NJ: New Century, 1983.

————. *The McDougall Program: Twelve Days to Dynamic Health.* New York: NAL Books, 1990.

Moran, V. *Compassion the Ultimate Ethic: An Exploration of Veganism.* Malaga, NJ: American Vegan Society, 2nd rev. ed. 1991.

————. *The Love-Powered Diet: When Willpower Is Not Enough.* San Rafael, CA: New World Library, 1992.

Robbins, J. *Diet for a New America.* Walpole, NH: Stillpoint Publishing, 1987. A most important book that can be recommended to anyone.

Organizations

The American Vegan Society, Box H, Malaga, NJ 08328. Offers support and information on vegan diet and life-style.

EarthSave, P.O. Box 949, Felton, CA 95018-0949. Environmental organization whose primary purpose is to encourage widespread adoption of the vegan diet.

The Yoga of Eating
by Omraam Mikhael Aivanhov

Eating is a magic rite during which the food becomes transformed into health, force, love, light. Observe yourself, if you eat in a state of anger, agitation, discontent, you will be left with a bitter taste in your mouth all day; you will feel nervous and tense, and, if there are difficult problems to be solved, you will be negative in your reactions; your decisions will lack fairness and comprehension; you will not be generous enough to make concessions. It will do no good to justify yourself, "It isn't my fault, I am so nervous, I simply cannot help it!" and then swallow some medicine or other to try and calm yourself (which will do no good either). To improve your nervous system, you must learn to eat properly. . . .

Learning that we can trust the creative energy of Life itself enables us to relax more and more because we know we don't have to make things happen by the force of our will.

SWAMI CHETANANANDA

While you eat you should think of the food with love, for that will make it open its treasures to you. . . . When the sun warms the flowers, they open up; when it disappears, they close. If you love food, if you eat it lovingly, it will open and exhale a fragrance for you and give you the etheric particles you are looking for. . . .

During meals you can develop your mind and your heart and also your will, since to acquire the habit of making restrained, deliberate, harmonious gestures, you are using willpower! When you feel nervous, seize the next mealtime as the opportunity to calm yourself, chew very slowly and be careful of every gesture: in a few minutes you will be calm again and at peace. . . .

The day is coming when nutrition will be considered the best of all yogas in spite of not having been mentioned before now. . . . It is the easiest yoga to learn; all creatures practise it unconsciously! . . .

Begin today to make your meals a time for spiritual work, the work that is so necessary, so indispensable. . . .

If we know how to listen, food speaks to us. Food is condensed light and sound, but if your thoughts are busy elsewhere, you cannot hear the 'voice' of the light. . . .

OVERCOMING EATING DISORDERS
BY GRETCHEN ROSE NEWMARK

The behaviors of eating disorders—binge eating (followed by purging, fasting, or excessive exercise) and rigid food restriction—constitute a kind of maladaptive ritual that brings a familiar, though painful, comfort to those who have come to rely on that ritual in order to cope. A hatha yoga class can replace a self-destructive ritual with a healthful one, particularly if the instructor includes the same or similar asanas in each class.

People who binge-eat often report a meditative quality in the repetitive, mindless quality of their eating. Unfortunately, many of them are too agitated to sit still in meditation. At the end of a yoga class, however, they can often relax and experience a meditative state that is much deeper and more fulfilling than the one induced by binging.

Yoga is a teacher of paradox. On the one hand, we must learn to *control* our impulses to get up and "do something" while we are seated in one of the yogic postures, and we must patiently await the signs of the body's progress. We learn that the body has its own rhythms and that it will sometimes unfold in ways that are beyond our conscious control or understanding.

Most people with eating disorders are seriously cut off from their body's signals—hunger and satiety, fatigue, satisfaction, sensual pleasure, even pain. Learning to let yourself eat when you are hungry and stop when you are full is one step toward letting go of binge eating or food restricting—as is learning to heed your body's requests for rest, pleasure, or attention. Becoming aware of how your body feels in a yoga pose helps to reawaken your sense of how your body communicates with you. I can still hear my first yoga teacher saying softly, "Just be still and *feel* it!" That simple reminder taught me so much: it was the first time I could remember paying attention to my body without trying to judge or change it.

Also, if you have problems with eating, you probably have difficulty dealing effectively with stress (or even knowing when you are stressed) because the obsession with eating masks signals of anxiety. The breathing, the muscle relaxation, and the focusing effect of yoga are all powerful teachers of "stress management." You can do head and neck rolls at your desk, or deep breathing when you feel pressured at a meeting. You can learn to calm anxiety by turning your attention inward and stilling the mind. Wherever you go, you can take with you the asanas that bring you peace and calm.

Remember, if you have the features of an eating disorder, you will probably have feelings of self-hatred which you will focus on your body. Whether of normal weight, emaciated, or overweight, a person with an eating disorder will see her body as an obstacle to getting what she wants from life. Her "fat" stomach, thighs, or whatever part she feels bad about becomes the object of her hatred and shame. Yoga teaches that the body is so much more than an object to be judged by its outward appearance. Yoga can awaken an understanding of the body as an extension of the mind—as a source of sensual pleasure, a spiritual home, a living, breathing entity that deserves love, acceptance, and appreciation. An instructor who emphasizes treating the body with affection and care can help speed this awakening.

Positive suggestion is another powerful way that hatha yoga can help you free yourself of an eating disorder. Milton Erickson, who pioneered the creative use of hypnosis in psychotherapy, pointed out that we are often in a "hypnotic" state even when not in an induced trance. We are most open to suggestion, whether positive or negative, when we are relaxed yet focused—the state of mind we cultivate in hatha yoga. You can take advantage of that focused, relaxed, trancelike state to allow positive, direct suggestions from your instructor or yourself to penetrate

The Body Is a Wise Organism
JACK SCHWARZ

deep into your subconscious mind. Your teacher might say something like, "Feel the energy reaching every cell, healing deep within you," or, "In Shavasana (Corpse Pose), sink into the floor and let it support you; feel yourself a part of all that is, safe and secure."

Or you can repeat positive affirmations like, "I find my desire to eat extra food gradually slipping away, as I feel more and more fulfilled and satisfied inside my body." Such affirmations—for example, "My body is exactly as it should be," or "My body is strong, supple, and secure"— also go well with certain asanas. Let your mind embrace these suggestions and make them yours, replacing negative thoughts and destructive self-talk. Getting better involves changing your automatic subconscious thoughts, and a hatha yoga class or a session on your own offers you a good opportunity to contact that part of yourself.

In Supine Toe-to-Head Pose (Supta Padangushthasana), Grace notices that her classmate has managed to get her leg closer to her head than she has. What is worse, to her competitive mind, is that the last time she did this asana, she was more flexible. Grace brings to class another predictable feature of eating disorders—her extremely competitive nature, her drive for perfection. She can never measure up to her own exacting standards, and by the time she has reached one goal, she is unable to enjoy it because she has already fixed on the next.

In my work I stress the noncompetitive nature of yoga, so much a contrast from the norm in our society. In yoga you don't need to compete with anyone, not even yourself. You can treat your body as though it were brand new to you, as yet untried in its ability to stretch, strengthen, and move. Let it surprise you, let it set its own limits, watch how it varies from session to session. Grace began to see her body, the focus of her competitiveness and self-hatred, as a process of unfolding, perfect just as it is. From it she could learn limits, rather than trying to impose limits of her own based on what she thought it ought to do.

Hatha yoga has such a deep effect on so many aspects of a person's being that it is a natural adjunct to counseling in the treatment of eating disorders, which are so complex and multifaceted by nature. Some clients are not attracted to yoga; to them I suggest another outlet, such as t'ai chi ch'uan, dance, art work, or music. The slow, passive styles of hatha yoga, which emphasize a receptive, meditative attitude, are effective in teaching people with eating disorders to *feel* emotions and urges, to heed them or let them pass, and to accept them completely. The more powerful, active forms of yoga are helpful in teaching a sense of personal power, direction, and effectiveness.

In my own experience and in my work with clients, I have found that the lessons learned from hatha yoga unfold gradually, mirroring the usual pace of counseling, where lasting results take time. During my first yoga class I noticed an immediate sense of relief and peace—and clients I have worked with have had similar experiences. Nevertheless, people are slow to make actual changes in eating or purging behaviors. For me, although I found hatha yoga deeply satisfying, I did not realize until years later, when I began to work with eating disorders professionally, how helpful yoga had been for me. Lessons learned in the "head" in counseling are often learned simultaneously in the "body" in yoga. Awareness gained in one stimulates awareness in the other.

Hatha yoga seems to be effective in the treatment of a variety of disorders because it allows us to feel our minds, bodies, and spirits in unison and to attend to their needs. Too little is still known about what works in the treatment of eating disorders, and there is no literature at this time that documents the effects of hatha yoga. However, I believe that hatha yoga has the potential to help us discover inner resources that make it easier to live life free of weight and food obsessions and that enhance counseling and other forms of treatment.

RESOURCES

Books

Cauwels, J. M. *Bulimia: The Binge-Purge Compulsion.* New York: Double-day, 1983.

Chernin, K. *The Obsession: Reflections on the Tyranny of Slenderness.* New York: Harper & Row, 1981.

Levenkron, S. *The Best Little Girl in the World.* New York: Warner Books, 1979.

Squire, S. *The Slender Balance.* New York: G. P. Putnam's Sons, 1983.

Woodman, M. *Addiction to Perfection.* New York: Inner City Books, 1982.

Periodicals

Anorexia Nervosa and Related Eating Disorders (ANRED) Newsletter, P.O. Box 5102, Eugene, OR 97405. This monthly newsletter offers locations of professionally led groups for people with eating disorders as well as practical articles written by people with eating disorders, therapists, nutritionists, and others.

Organizations

National Association of Anorexia Nervosa and Associated Disorders, Inc., Box 271, Highland Park, IL 60035. The Association provides general information on eating disorders and self-help groups in the United States.

TIPS FOR HEALTHY NUTRITION

1. Increase fruit, vegetables, and whole grains in your diet. Ideally, become a vegetarian.

2. Reduce processed foods, which contain additives and preservatives that have little nutritional value and in the long run have a toxic effect on the body.

3. Reduce your consumption of fats to no more than 20–30 percent of your daily calories.

4. Reduce your intake of sugar and sugar-loaded foods.

5. Reduce your intake of salt and overly salty foods.

6. Eliminate caffeine from your diet, whether in coffee or chocolate.

7. Drink plenty of pure water.

8. Don't eat when you are stressed-out or aggravated. Wait until you are calm again.

9. Prepare your meals so they look inviting.

10. Eat consciously, with enjoyment.

11. Don't overeat.

12. One day a week do a fruit juice or vegetable juice fast, which will help cleanse your system.

PART TWO

TRANSCENDING THE MIND: RAJA YOGA

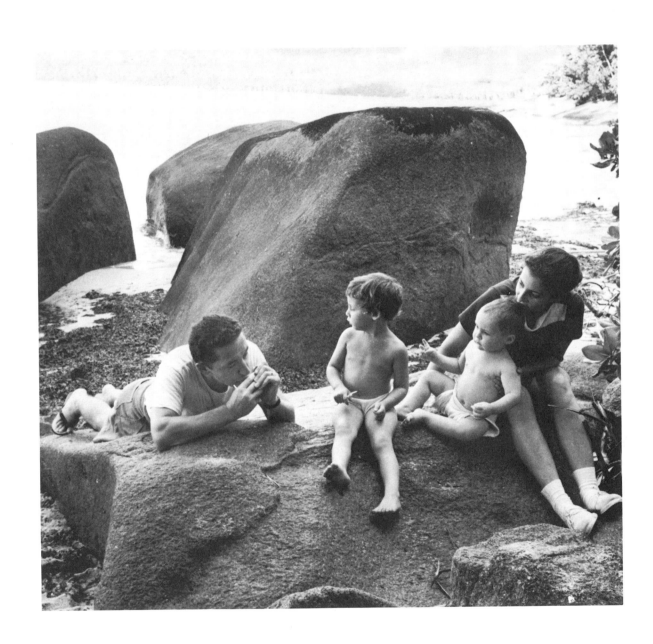

SIX

Relaxation and Well-Being

In our Western culture we tend to be addicted to stress, and stress is the primary cause of a wide range of degenerative diseases. To prevent unnecessary illness, we must learn to consciously relax. Relaxation is in fact at the very base of all yoga practice. This chapter explains why relaxation is important, and how to go about relaxing. It also looks at the healing process and the attitudes that you must cultivate to promote balance and health in your life.

Letting go a little improves life. Letting go a lot brings happiness and joy.

JIM MCGREGOR

FROM STRESS TO SUPERCONSCIOUSNESS

A certain amount of tension is natural to all living processes. Tension is inherent in nature itself. We see it in the atomic nucleus and in the cosmos at large, where the mysterious force of gravity holds together entire galaxies revolving around a common central point.

By contrast, when viewed from a higher spiritual perspective, stress is largely a self-destructive psychological state. It is a condition indicative of an individual who tends to be at odds with himself or herself, and with life as such. This is, of course, true for most of us who live ordinary lives and who only occasionally experience what psychologist Mihaly Csikszentmihalyi calls "flow." He explains:

'Flow' is the way people describe their state of mind when consciousness is harmoniously ordered, and they want to pursue whatever they are doing for its own sake. [1]

When we "flow," our experience is devoid of either boredom or anxiety, and we are spontaneous, confident, courageous, and centered.

When we experience stress, however, we tend to be self-conscious and full of doubt. Some people deal with stress more creatively than others. But beyond the stress syndrome, and our attempts to cope with it, lies the joyous experience of flow, or attunement to reality.

One of the physical correlates of stress is chronically high blood pressure, "hypertension." Approximately 20 percent of Americans reportedly suffer from hypertension. Other widespread symptoms of stress are chronic headaches, irritable bowel syndrome, and ulcers.

We can understand stress as a mismanagement of our time and energy. Instead of living in the present, which is possible only when we are inwardly still and centered, we worry about the future and regret the past. Our worries reduce our sense of available time in the present, and we feel we don't have enough time to do what we want to accomplish. This causes us to be less efficient in dealing with life's tasks and problems. This, in turn, causes us to worry more, so we try to cram as many things as possible into the day, without really winning the battle.

Our emotional pressure raises our blood pressure, and so on, and we become nervous, overactive, and unable to relax, sleep, and recuperate. We are locked into a vicious circle.

From a profound philosophical point of view, stress can be characterized as a state of the ego par excellence. The ego feels it never has enough time to express itself. It fears its own inevitable demise and looks upon time as its arch enemy, trying to beat time by gluttonously devouring a multitude of experiences. Of course, time does not stand still, and experiences do not finally fulfill us. Our search for happiness and fulfillment is, therefore, always frustrated.

When we transcend the ego, we leave behind stress. That is, when we stop clinging to the limited sense of who we are (or are not), when we relax our attachment to what we deem as "I," "me," and "mine," we simultaneously undo the tension the ego creates. The ego is like a rock projecting out of a meandering river. It creates resistance and causes the otherwise peaceful flow of the water to form eddies and cross currents (our familiar egoic problems).

As we let go of our ego, we gradually discover Being, or our innermost Self, which has all the time in the world and has no concerns. The Self is superconscious, that is, it is not boxed in, confined to a body, a particular brain, or memory.

Yoga is a progressive path of ego-transcendence through relaxing our self-imposed boundaries, our home-spun illusions that we are identical to the body and objective things. Yoga proceeds to ever deeper levels of relaxing the ego.

We have lost our way in time. More and more, time has become a commodity, a resource to be used and hoarded, traded and exploited.

DIANA HUNT AND
PAM HAIT

Raja yoga, the "royal yoga," seeks to accomplish this task by controlling the mind directly. Ordinarily, the mind is a busy chatterbox, with thoughts piling upon thoughts, fleeting emotions piling upon fleeting emotions. Through concentration, the practitioner of raja yoga endeavors to still the mind, to bring harmony to the inner environment. But unlike ordinary concentration, which we engage in when doing intellectual work, for instance, yogic concentration is possible only in conjunction with complete physical relaxation. Somatic relaxation is the other side of the spiritual letting-go of the ego's stranglehold.

Yogic concentration (dharana) is a state of creative tension, of one-pointedness, in which we get in touch with the deeper aspects of the body-mind. Concentration leads to meditation, and meditation is the ground from which the seed of superconscious ecstasy, present in all of us, may burst into full flower. When the Self's innate delight manifests in us, we experience the peace that passeth all understanding. In that moment we are no longer subject to anxiety about life or the fear of death. Life reveals itself to be a playful drama in which we, as self-transcending persons, are called to joyously participate.

We are free to be at peace with ourselves and others, and also with nature.

THOMAS MERTON

RESOURCES

Books

Easwaran, E. *Meditation: A Simple 8-Point Program for Translating Spiritual Ideals into Daily Life.* Tomales, CA: Nilgiri Press, 2nd ed., 1991.

Naranjo, C. *How to Be: Meditation in Spirit and Practice.* Los Angeles: J. P. Tarcher, 1990.

Swami Ajaya. *Yoga Psychology: A Practical Guide to Meditation.* Honesdale, PA: Himalayan International Institute, 1976.

Swami Sivananda. *Concentration and Meditation.* Shivanandanagar, India: Divine Life Society, 1975.

Swami Vivekananda. *Raja Yoga.* New York: Ramakrishna-Vivekananda Center, 1982.

THE RELAXATION RESPONSE AND BEYOND
BY PEGGY R. GILLESPIE

Even when life appears to be going well, stress can build up, wearing down even the healthiest among us. Hatha yoga can make a big difference, of course, but yoga alone may not counteract all the debilitating effects of stress: sore muscles, headaches, chest pains, back spasms, heart palpitations, skin problems, and emotional problems such as depression, poor concentration, and chronic anxiety. Ultimately, if left unchecked, stress can lead to serious illness, and even death.

What Is Stress?

There is no educational requirement or aptitude necessary to experience the Relaxation Response. Just as each of us experiences anger, contentment, and excitement, each has the capacity to experience the Relaxation Response.

HERBERT BENSON

Stress, in itself, is neither good nor bad—it is simply the way our bodies respond to any change or challenge, big or small, positive or negative. When we go from a warm room into the cold air, run two blocks to catch a bus, have an argument with a friend, get a raise, get fired, get married, or get divorced, we experience some of the effects of stress.

The physical changes that indicate the presence of stress—tight shoulders, clammy hands, headache, upset stomach, tight chest, and so forth—result from the arousal of many bodily systems. This state of arousal, called the *fight-or-flight response,* is a natural and instinctive reaction to a life-threatening situation.

Whenever we perceive an actual or anticipated event to be threatening, our physiological response is basically the same: The brain stimulates the adrenal glands to release adrenaline-related hormones into the bloodstream. The results include the following:

- Increased heart rate

- Elevated blood pressure

- Rapid, shallow breathing

- Release of stored energy from the liver into the bloodstream

- Dilation of pupils to let in more light

- Heightening of all senses

- Tensing of muscles for movement or protective actions

- Activation of blood-clotting mechanisms

- Shutdown of digestive processes; blood diverted to muscles and brain

- Constriction of blood flow to the extremities

- Sweating

Once the immediate threat is gone, the body lets go, the stress hormones begin to recede, and we are left feeling drained and tired. Eventually, the body returns to its normal state of equilibrium.

In the 1930s Dr. Hans Selye began to do research showing the results of sustained physiological arousal on living organisms. In 1956 he published his landmark work, *The Stress of Life*, which concludes that when the source of stress is prolonged or undefined, or when several sources exist at once, an individual may not return to a normal mental or physiological baseline. Instead, he or she will continue to manifest potentially damaging stress reactions and symptoms; ultimately, Selye found, prolonged and uninterrupted stress leads to complete exhaustion, and finally death.

Stress serves as the cardinal example of how mind, brain, and body interact.

MICHAEL S. GAZZANIGA

Medical Treatment of Stress-Related Disorders

Western medicine in the twentieth century has emphasized technological advancement. In recent decades, old-fashioned family doctors familiar with the life histories of their patients have all but disappeared, replaced by specialists trained to examine and treat one area of a patient's body. Hospitals have become big businesses, medical costs have skyrocketed, and health insurance plans cover disease treatments but refuse to pay for most preventive health care.

Until recently, medical intervention for the treatment of stress-related disorders has relied almost exclusively on medications for symptom control. For the common disorders diagnosed as muscular or nervous tension, 144 million new prescriptions were written in just one recent year, many for drugs with unpleasant side effects. In fact, three of the best-selling drugs in the U.S. are for stress-related conditions: an ulcer medication (Tagamet), a hypertension drug (Inderal), and a central nervous system depressant (Valium).

Fortunately, in the past twenty years, there has been a growing interest in non-pharmacological methods for preventing and healing diseases that have been demonstrated to have emotional components. The overwhelming evidence in support of a relationship between stress and disease has forced medicine to begin to turn to more preventive approaches. As researchers have recognized the role of the mind in creating certain illnesses, they also have realized that the treatment of these diseases must involve the body-mind connection.

Another factor leading to the emergence of more "holistic" approaches to medicine has been the increasing interest, in the past twenty-five years, in Eastern philosophies and healing practices. Among those

Stress causes dramatic reductions in the ability to think coherently and creatively, and to perform movements requiring skill and dexterity.

MICHAEL HUTCHISON

who have looked to the East have been physicians, psychologists, and other scientists who have discovered that ancient medical techniques differ radically from modern Western methods. These health professionals have been exposed to sophisticated Oriental systems like Chinese medicine and Ayurveda, which emphasize prevention of disease by balancing physical, emotional, and spiritual energies.

They have also observed meditators and yoga practitioners who can consciously control such bodily functions as heart rate and blood pressure, previously considered by Western science to be beyond human voluntary control. A common factor seen in all Asian medical traditions has been the emphasis on the treatment of the whole person—mind, body, and spirit.

At the height of this interest in Eastern approaches to body and mind, an Indian guru, Maharishi Mahesh Yogi, came to the West and persuaded millions of Americans to try a form of mantra meditation known as Transcendental Meditation (TM) as a way to increase physical well-being and mental functioning. The time was obviously ripe: TM became the first form of Eastern spiritual technology to gain widespread acceptance in this country. Soon IBM executives and Bell Telephone operators were extolling the benefits of meditation. Coffee breaks became 20-minute TM breaks. And Maharishi's message is still reverberating.

Meditation was catapulted into the medical mainstream by the publication, in 1975, of *The Relaxation Response* by Harvard cardiologist Herbert Benson. Convinced by practitioners of TM to study the effects of this meditation practice on human physiology, Benson discovered that one does not have to become a guru or a mystic to learn to control blood pressure, body temperature, respiration rate, heart rate, and oxygen consumption.

His experiments revealed that many people were able to achieve the same results using this simple form of meditation. Benson believed that the outcome of this type of meditation was the ability to elicit what he called the "relaxation response," the exact opposite of the fight-or-flight response. Benson's work paved the way for further studies of the use of self-regulatory, non-invasive techniques in the prevention and cure of stress-related illness.

As holistic medicine has gained wider acceptance, new departments of pain control, behavioral and preventive medicine, and stress reduction have begun to sprout right within the halls of otherwise traditional hospitals and medical clinics. Even the AMA has recommended the use of relaxation techniques as a first step before medication for the treatment of borderline hypertension, and more and more people are seeking such treatments on their own, despite the skepticism of their more conservative physicians. TM and the "relaxation response" are only two of the many different relaxation techniques offered. As a potential consumer, you might well find yourself wondering, "How can I sort out the most effective treatment for me?"

Let me make clear from the outset that there is no perfect technique that will miraculously take your stress away—and anyone who promises such results is like the proverbial snake oil salesman. Along with the positive benefits of holistic medicine have come quacks and opportunists. If you are seeking a program to help you reduce your stress, it is best to be as cautious as you would in choosing a physician. Attend a class as an observer, if possible, before paying out lots of money. And, above all, enjoy the program. If you find yourself dreading your stress reduction class, you can be sure you aren't in the right place. Stress reduction, when taught well, should be an exhilarating experience.

Learning to relax and quiet the mind can make you feel better, function better, and maintain better health.

FRANCES VAUGHAN

Choosing a Suitable Relaxation Technique

All relaxation techniques require that you assume a high level of responsibility. Don't expect change to come easily. And, above all, don't expect your stress level to diminish magically to zero after an eight-week course. Remember, it took you years to become as tense as you are. It will take dedication and patience to learn how to become more relaxed. If you have practiced hatha yoga, you know the kind of effort and perseverance that are required to overcome years of negative physical conditioning.

If you have never engaged in a regular psychophysical discipline, you may be surprised at how long it can take you to develop the ability to relax deeply. In any case, don't lose heart. The importance of relaxation techniques in reducing stress and increasing immune system function has been well documented, so your patience will be well rewarded.

Many people believe that relaxation is the exact opposite of tension. They picture themselves lying around the house or office as useless as a limp strand of linguine, unable to move, think, or act decisively. Jack H., a lawyer, said, "Sure I want to get rid of my colitis, but I also need to appear strong and confident, especially at work. I certainly don't want to become known as a space cadet or some cross-legged, do-nothing yogi mumbling weird chants under my breath." Jack assumed that being relaxed required a complete change of personality. His misconceptions and fears prevented him from learning some basic ways of being in the world in a calm and energetic manner.

Relaxation can occur on many levels, from the absence of noticeable tension in the mind and body to the experience of deep inner states of psychological and spiritual peace. The following widely used, well-researched techniques induce relaxation primarily at the physiological level. Physiological relaxation is characterized by changes in the body that are opposite in almost all respects to the fight-or-flight response: the slowing down of breath and heart rates, a decrease in oxygen consumption, and the lowering or stabilization of blood pressure. In a separate table I have listed what I perceive to be the advantages and disadvantages of using each technique as the basis of a stress reduction program.

ADVANTAGES AND DISADVANTAGES OF VARIOUS STRESS REDUCTION TECHNIQUES

Technique	Advantages	Disadvantages
TM/Relaxation Response	Simple to do; instructions readily available. Health benefits scientifically proven, well publicized.	Repetitive; may become boring. Daily practice may be difficult to maintain. Relationship between regular practice and ability to cope with stress may not be readily apparent.
Progressive Relaxation	Simple to learn, provides immediate feedback. Requires no special equipment or environment.	Cannot be used by those unable to move or use their muscles. Repetitive; may become boring. Requires frequent practice. Relationship between regular practice and ability to cope with stress may not be readily apparent.
Autogenic Training	Symptom oriented; works well with specific problems. Instructions simple, easy to follow. Requires no special equipment or environment.	Learning requires frequent contact with trained practitioner. Repetitive; may become boring. Requires frequent practice. Relationship between regular practice and ability to cope with stress may not be readily apparent.

Technique	Advantages	Disadvantages
Biofeedback	Provides immediate feedback, sense of control over one's bodily processes. With proper training, equipment eventually becomes unnecessary. Effectiveness scientifically proven, well publicized.	Equipment and training can be quite expensive. Requires frequent visits to therapist's office. Some people may be unable to transfer learning to daily lives, may become dependent on equipment. Failure to achieve desired effect may lead to heightened anxiety and low self-esteem.
Visualization	Many people find it easy to learn. May have positive effects on immune system function. Emphasis on will and responsibility lend a heightened sense of control. Requires no special equipment or environment.	Some people find visualization difficult or impossible to learn, which may increase anxiety. Effectiveness not well substantiated. Does not prevent person from repeatedly triggering stress reaction.
Breathing Exercises	Easy to learn; training inexpensive. Can be used during daily activities as reminder to relax.	Repetitive; may become boring. Increases awareness of stress reactivity without fostering understanding of causes.
Hatha Yoga	Deep physiological relaxation; stretches muscles and strengthens body. Appeals to people who find meditation too passive. Can be done at home or in inexpensive class. Interesting variety of poses; not likely to become boring. Can be adapted to those with physical problems.	Cannot be used by those unable to move or use their muscles. Does not appeal to those who do not like to do any form of exercise. Competitiveness and goal orientation may defeat purpose as relaxation technique. Requires frequent practice. Relationship between regular practice and ability to cope with stress may not be readily apparent.

TM and/or the Relaxation Response

A sound, word, or phrase is repeated, silently or audibly, for 15 to 20 minutes twice a day. The purpose of this repetition is to divert attention from the constant flow of sensory input and thought processes. The meditator sits or lies in a comfortable position to eliminate muscle strain and physical tension; a quiet environment is recommended to prevent unwanted interruptions.

Progressive Relaxation

Learning to feel and control muscular tension is the basis of an effective and widely used relaxation method first described in 1938 by Dr. Edmund Jacobson. He noticed that it was easier to tense a muscle group first, then use the tension as a platform from which to experience relaxation. His method depends on systematically tensing and relaxing muscle groups throughout the body, starting with the feet.

Progressive relaxation originally required months of daily practice, one to two hours a day, and Jacobson claimed that this regimen could successfully treat anxiety disorders and a variety of other illnesses, including colitis and hypertension. In a recent study, progressive relaxation was helpful in decreasing blood pressure in a group of hypertensive patients. Modern clinicians have shortened the practice periods, making the technique more practical for everyday use.

Autogenic Training

This technique was invented in the 1890s by a German brain physiologist, Oskar Vogt, who observed that people could be taught to do self-hypnosis through a system of simple mental exercises. In 1905, psychiatrist Johannes Schultz continued Vogt's studies and found that, as patients' tension was relieved, they could learn to create sensations of warmth and heaviness in their arms and legs. The method was popularized by Schultz's colleague, Wolfgang Luthe, M.D., who also did extensive research.

During autogenic training, a patient sits or lies comfortably with her eyes closed and is asked to repeat silently a series of "standard phrases," e.g., "My breath is calm and regular" or "My hand feels warm and heavy." These phrases are intended to produce sensations of heaviness and warmth in the hands and feet, a slow and regular heartbeat, slow and regular breathing, and feelings of warmth in the abdomen and coolness in the forehead. Studies done in German laboratories have shown that autogenic training decreases heart rate, blood pressure, respiratory rate, and respiratory volume.

Biofeedback

Dr. Barbara Brown, noted biofeedback researcher, defines it as a "process or technique for learning voluntary control over automatic reflex-regulated body functions."[2] Biofeedback instruments monitor selected bodily functions, such as muscle tension, body temperature, brain waves, and skin conductivity, which are picked up by electrodes and transformed into visual or auditory signals. Any internal change instantly triggers an external signal, so that, when a patient is hooked up to the biofeedback equipment, she can continuously monitor her bodily functions and relaxation levels. Studies of the effectiveness of biofeedback have shown that a person who can actually see her heart rate change can learn to raise or lower it at will.

In the years since the discovery of biofeedback, the procedures have grown increasingly sensitive and capable of monitoring all types of physiological occurrences and displaying this feedback in a variety of forms, such as audible sounds, meter readings, and digital displays. In the West, biofeedback is probably the most well respected of the stress reduction techniques, as the results are easily measured, and research can be done in a scientifically acceptable manner.

For example, Elmer and Alyce Green of the Menninger Foundation conducted a series of experiments to test the effectiveness of autogenic training, both by itself and when reinforced by biofeedback. They learned that autogenic training alone was not nearly as effective as biofeedback alone, but that excellent results were obtained when the two methods were combined. According to the Biofeedback Society of America, specific treatment applications are currently considered promising for migraine headache, tension headache, neuromuscular reeducation following stroke, fecal incontinence, Reynaud's syndrome, certain forms of insomnia, and high blood pressure.

Visualization

This approach attempts to use the imagination to effect changes in the body. A person may be asked to consciously create mental images in order to alleviate or cure certain symptoms or diseases, such as warts, coronary artery disease, hypertension, eczema, ulcers, and even cancer. Some people have reported miraculous cures, which they partly or completely attribute to a daily period of visualization. This approach to stress reduction is almost always used in conjunction with another method of relaxation training, and its effectiveness is very difficult to prove conclusively. The anecdotal evidence can be persuasive, however, and numerous books on visualization have been published, reflecting its growing popularity.

The body can feel completely at ease and natural every moment. Just let it.

EUGENE GENDLIN

Breathing Exercises

Throughout the centuries, breathing exercises have been an integral part of mental, physical, and spiritual development in Eastern cultures. Thoracic (chest) breathing is directly related to the activation of the fight-or-flight arousal mechanism; hence, training patients in diaphragmatic breathing can help them learn to prevent stress reactivity and to facilitate a quicker return to a balanced state after a stress reaction. Exercises can retrain a person to breathe correctly in a relaxed, calm manner. They can also provide the same benefits as concentration meditation practices like TM, because, instead of using a mantra, the practitioner focuses on the sensations of the breath. These exercises include various methods of controlling the breath as well as ways to observe the natural flow of the diaphragmatic breath.

Hatha Yoga

In the past twenty years, yoga has grown quite popular throughout the Western world. Some instructors emphasize its benefits in healing and preventing back problems. Others stress its role as a spiritual discipline that helps to create heightened levels of consciousness. But most will agree that yoga has an unparalleled ability to energize and relax the body through its slow, deliberate movements performed with concentration and precision. There are even courses designed especially for elderly people, who have found that yoga has relieved symptoms of bursitis, arthritis, and muscular tension, while increasing strength and overall energy levels.

Understanding the Causes of Stress

Most reputable stress reduction classes combine several of these modalities to increase the probability of a client's success and enjoyment. Definite physiological benefits have been shown to occur when any form of relaxation technique is practiced. Nevertheless, many experts in the field, myself among them, believe that in order to begin to manage stress in a profound, life-altering manner, one must first understand the basic causes of the stress reaction.

If we do not understand and uproot the causes of stress, we may be unpleasantly surprised to find that TM, progressive relaxation, biofeedback, even hatha yoga, are only stop-gap measures, which do not help that much when we are deluged by the crises and minor hassles of daily life.

In *Freedom from Stress*, Dr. Philip Nuernberger writes: "In terms of stress management, it is true that a consistent practice of relaxation and physical exercises will modify or alleviate stress, but they will not eliminate the stress-inducing patterns in the mind. Doing only relaxation and physical exercises is like putting out a fire—only to come back and find it burning again. It is more efficient to remove the conditions which create the fire than it is to continually have to put the fire out. In other words, it is much simpler and more effective to understand the subtle mental/emotional origins of stress, and then to alter or remove them, than it is to continually rescue the body and mind from stress."[3]

Relaxation Alone Is Not Enough

Any of the popular relaxation methods could help us calm down and think more clearly. But they are only a beginning. A deeper level of stress management must not only alleviate symptoms, as drugs can also do, but also help us to develop insight into our mental patterns and help our conditioned stress reactions. To go this deep, stress management must involve self-discovery, in addition to relaxation exercises.

Such sweeping attitudinal changes would seem to require in-depth, individual psychotherapy. But therapy, though it can be extremely helpful in the resolution of stress issues, can also be extremely expensive, unavailable, or threatening to some. To help clients get to know themselves on the deepest levels, Dr. Jon Kabat Zinn, director of the innovative Stress Reduction and Relaxation Program (SR & RP) at the University of Massachusetts Medical Center, decided to use Buddhist mindfulness meditation practice as the basis of his approach. According to Kabat-Zinn, mindfulness occasions a level of relaxation that is deeper and longer lasting than the purely physiological level described earlier.

The Benefits of Mindfulness

The practice of traditional mindfulness meditation consists of two basic forms. Meditators begin by developing their powers of concentration through mindfulness of the breath on the inhalation and exhalation. As their ability to concentrate increases, they are taught to use this skill to develop the second form, which is the observation of all aspects of the body and mind: sensations, sights, sounds, thoughts, and emotions.

Meditators are instructed to return their attention to the present moment whenever they notice that their mind is lost in thought. By bringing detailed awareness to the body, they begin to see how patterns of physical tension may be creating unnecessary pain or other unpleasant symptoms. By bringing detailed awareness to thought, they begin to see how patterns—of fear, reactivity, craving, holding on to

Pledge yourself to remain serene throughout the day whatever happens; to be a living example of serenity; to radiate serenity.

ROBERTO ASSAGIOLI

123

self-images and opinions, refusing to accept the impermanence of life itself—create suffering in the mind. Once meditators are able to see that their reactions to the stressors in life are habitual and conditioned, they can begin to move from being victims of circumstances to a more powerful and hopeful position where change is possible.

When we develop insight into our behavior, the personal experience of such insight can motivate profound internal and external changes. Such strong inner motivation is absolutely essential if a patient is to be successful in a self-regulatory program. Even more important, mindfulness practice is not limited to periods of formal practice; it is meant to become a way of life. The ability to observe our mind and body with a degree of non-judgmental detachment becomes an inseparable part of us. We cannot discard it as we might discard a visualization process, an asana practice, or the recitation of a mantra. As awareness permeates every activity and every communication, we are able to shift from "automatic pilot" to a more spontaneous, joyful appreciation and acceptance of life as it unfolds.

RESOURCES

Although stress management programs are available nationwide through medical clinics, HMOs, hospitals, business offices, and YMCAs, as well as privately with therapists who are stress management experts, many programs emphasize physiological relaxation techniques rather than the development of "deep inner relaxation." If you cannot find a program like the one at the University of Massachusetts, which uses mindfulness as its core practice, try supplementing your local classes with the following books and tapes.

Books

Bloomfield, H., et al. *TM: How Meditation Can Reduce Stress.* New York: Dell, 1975. A comprehensive introduction to Transcendental Meditation (TM) and the medical and psychological studies done on this system of meditation.

Borysenko, J. *Minding the Body, Mending the Mind.* New York: Bantam, 1987. Practical exercises based on the methods developed at the University of Massachusetts. The author describes her experiences in helping to establish a stress reduction clinic at a Harvard teaching hospital.

Gillespie, P. R., and L. Bechtel. *Less Stress in 30 Days: An Integrated Approach for Relaxation.* New York: Signet Books, 1987. Follows a comprehensive, day-by-day stress reduction plan based on our work at the

University of Massachusetts Medical Center and the University of Massachusetts, Amherst.

Goleman, D., and T. Bennet-Goleman. *The Relaxed Body Book.* New York: Doubleday, 1986. Exercises for relaxing the body using mindfulness meditation and physical techniques.

Audiotapes

The tapes used at the University of Massachusetts Stress Reduction and Relaxation Program are available from Stress Reduction Tapes, University of Massachusetts Medical Center, 55 Lake Avenue, North Worcester, MA 01605.

Le Shan, Lawrence, *How to Meditate;* Goleman, D., *The Art of Meditation;* Young, S., *Five Classic Meditations.* All three are available from Audio Renaissance Tapes, 5858 Wilshire Blvd., Los Angeles, CA 90036.

TURNING STRESS INTO STRENGTH: TIPS FOR STRESS REDUCTION
BY JOEL LEVEY, PH.D., AND MICHELLE LEVEY, M.A.

Life's myriad changes often lead to an accumulation of stress. Here is a compendium of simple, common-sense strategies for transforming mental and physical tension into energy creatively and effectively expressed. None of these strategies are new. Many will be familiar to you, but we often need to be reminded. Circle the ones you'd like to remember more often. Then add your own to the list.

- Take time to be alone on a regular basis, to listen to your heart, check your intentions, re-evaluate your goals and your activities.

- Simplify your life! Start eliminating the trivia.

- Take deep, slow breaths frequently, especially while on the phone, in the car, or waiting for something or someone. Use any opportunity to relax and revitalize yourself.

- Plan to do something each day that brings you joy, something that you love to do, something just for you.

- When you're concerned about something, talk it over with someone you trust, or write down your feelings.

- Say No when asked to do something you really don't want to do. Read a book on assertiveness if you have trouble doing this in a firm but kind way.

- Remember to use helpful clichés such as, "In a hundred years, who will know the difference?" "What doesn't weaken us, makes us stronger," or "Whether you think you can or you think you can't, you're right."

- Exercise regularly!

- Remember, it takes less energy to get an unpleasant task done "right now" than to worry about it all day.

- Take time to be with nature, people, music, and children. Even in the city, noticing the seasonal changes of the sky or watching people's faces can be a good harmonizer.

- Practice consciously doing one thing at a time, keeping your mind focused on the present. Do whatever you're doing more slowly, more intentionally, and with more awareness and respect.

- Choose not to waste your precious present life on guilt about the past or concern for the future.

- Learn a variety of relaxation techniques and practice at least one regularly.

- Let your eyes be soft and relaxed.

- When you find yourself repeatedly angry in similar situations, ask yourself, "What can I learn from this?" Anyone or anything that can make you angry is showing you how you yourself let yourself be controlled by expectations of how someone or something should be. When we accept others, ourselves and situations for what they are, we become more effective in influencing them to change in the way that we'd like them to.

- Practice stress-reducing communications: Clarify what you hear by paraphrasing (e.g., "I understand you to be saying . . .") and active listening. Use "I want" instead of "I need," and "I choose to" rather than "I have to." Feel the difference in your mental attitude and your body when you do this.

- Become more aware of the demands you place on yourself, your environment, and on others to be different from how they are at any moment. Demands are tremendous sources of stress.

- If your schedule is busy, prioritize your activities and do the most important ones first.

- When you read your mail, act on it immediately, don't put it off.

- Take frequent relaxation breaks.

- Carry a card with four or five personal affirmations written on it (e.g., "I am calm and relaxed," or "I am confident and capable of handling any situation").

- Organize your life to include time for fun, spontaneity, and open spaces. Set a realistic schedule allowing some transition time between activities. Eliminate unnecessary commitments.

- Smile and laugh more.

- Learn to delegate responsibility.

- Treat yourself to a massage, or learn to massage your own neck, shoulders, and feet.

- Monitor your intake of sugar, salt, caffeine, and alcohol.

- Create and maintain a personal support system—people with whom you can be "vulnerable."

- Seek out friends or professional help when you feel unable to cope.

- Be more kind to yourself and others.

- Appreciate the flow of change moment to moment. Welcome change as an opportunity and challenge to learn and grow.

- Watch clouds or waves on water. Listen to music or the sounds around you. Notice the silence between sounds and the space between objects and thoughts.

- When you notice you are stressed, smile tenderly to yourself, and breathe and let flow. Ahhh . . .

- Use your own distress to teach you to be more patient, caring, and compassionate toward yourself and others.

- Remember to stop and smell the flowers!

LOVE IS THE HEALER:
AN INTERVIEW WITH JOAN BORYSENKO
BY STEPHAN BODIAN

Conventional medicine generally attempts to heal the body; more holistic approaches address both the body and the mind. In your second book, Guilt Is the Teacher, Love Is the Lesson, *you seem to expand the domain of healing from the body-mind to the whole person, including the spiritual dimension.*

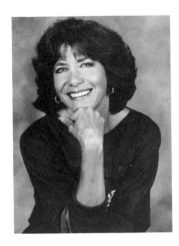

JOAN BORYSENKO

Psychology and medicine in this country don't have a place for the spiritual, for basic questions of meaning such as Who am I? or What is human life? After all, what can a person's belief system possibly have to do with their defense mechanisms, for instance, or their high blood pressure? As I began to listen to the stories of more and more patients, however, I began to have a very different point of view.

Martin Seligman, a psychologist at the University of Pennsylvania, has written a great deal about psychological pessimism. According to Seligman, psychological pessimists make three attributions when a "bad event" occurs: internal, global, and stable. Let's say you are a student who has just failed an algebra exam. If you are a psychological pessimist, you might say, "It's all my fault (internal). I'm a bad student, I mess up everything I do (global). And I'm always going to be like this (stable)." It's not just that you failed the exam because you had too many courses this term, or because the teacher wasn't that good, or because you hate algebra. It's because you're a hopeless good-for-nothing who is never going to change. You have this pervasive sense of what I've come to call unhealthy guilt. No matter what you do, it's never good enough. In my book I look at how we become psychological pessimists.

Do you suppose these people have an innate disposition to see things one way or another?

Their view of themselves correlates entirely with self-esteem. The higher the view they have of themselves, the more they see God as loving. The lower their self-esteem, the more self-punitive they are, the more they project a God in their own image.

This brings us back to stress and stress-related illness, where questions of meaning are of primary importance. Someone once asked Albert Einstein, "What is the most important question that we as human beings have to answer?" Einstein said, "It's simple. Is the universe a friendly place or not?" Now, we know for sure that bad things happen: people get sick and die, children starve, volcanoes erupt. In spite of that, many people believe in the sacred mystery of things. They believe that the force of love is operative and that, despite the uncertainty, we can still live rewarding, loving, happy lives. These people are spiritual optimists. Whereas if you are worried all the time that the world is an unsafe place or that you are being punished for your sins, it doesn't matter how much psychotherapy you do, or how much insight you have, or how much yoga or meditation you practice.

Many psychologists suggest that the predisposition to see the world as a negative, hostile place is learned very early, possibly even in the womb. How does one change in a radical way the experiences of early childhood?

First of all, I think one has to become conscious of them. Most of us don't give much thought to the meaning of things. For some people, their religious upbringing has been a bridge to the best in themselves and in other people. For other people, like myself, their religious tradition has been neither helpful nor injurious. But then there is a whole cadre of people out there who were damaged by their religious upbringing. Often they have turned off to it and said, "This is a pile of nonsense. I have no interest in it whatsoever." But it hasn't gone away. So the first task is to bring our awareness to what is going on inside us.

Once we have become aware of our beliefs, what next?

For one thing, there is a growing groundswell of support for spiritual optimism, even in the Judeo-Christian tradition. Then I also believe we are undergoing what Willis Harman has called a global mind change, from a metaphysics in which consciousness is seen as an attribute of the physical brain, to a metaphysics in which consciousness is primary and matter is derivative of consciousness. Once you have decided that consciousness is located in the brain, you have to conclude that consciousness ceases when the brain dies and that one person's thought cannot possibly affect another person at a distance. But Larry Dossey, in his book *Recovering the Soul*, makes the case that consciousness is nonlocal and can affect our health in a nonlocal way, that is, my thoughts can affect you at a distance in a way that is good for your health.

In my book I cite a well-known study by Randolph Byrd that made quite a splash a couple of years ago. Byrd was a cardiologist at San Francisco General Hospital who decided to do a study on the efficacy of prayer. He took 500 patients who had been admitted to the coronary intensive care unit, either for heart attack or to rule out heart attack, and he had them randomly assigned to a prayed-for and a not-prayed-for group. It was the pinnacle of controlled scientific research: a randomized double-blind study. None of the staff knew who was in which group so they couldn't preferentially give care to one group and not the other, and the subjects were chosen at random, so factors like sex, age, health, and demographics would balance out. Then he farmed out their names to prayer groups of various denominations around the country.

Man is not disturbed by things, but by his opinions about things.

GREEK PHILOSOPHER
EPICTETUS

When they broke the code at the end of the study, they found that indeed the prayed-for patients did significantly better on a number of measures. They got fewer infections, needed fewer antibiotics, got out of the hospital sooner. No one in the prayed-for group needed a respirator, whereas 16 or 17 of the others did. The differences were so significant that if prayer had been a drug, there would have been a run on the market for it. One well-known debunker of similar studies could find absolutely nothing wrong with this one. "Now I can truly say," he wrote, "that physicians should take out their pads and write prescriptions for prayer." There is no way to explain these results in terms of a brain generating consciousness in the body. The only way to explain it is that somehow the thoughts of one person can affect another person at a distance. Of course, for most of us this is just common sense.

There seems to be a tendency among people who get sick and are unable to cure themselves to feel guilty about it, as if they have failed in some way.

People will always prefer guilt over helplessness. No one wants to feel that they are completely powerless; they'd rather blame themselves, because in blame at least there's the sense that it's someone's fault. Why are bad things happening? We are still being punished for Eve's sin. If we are being punished, that means we are not powerless. If we follow certain moral precepts, we can be redeemed.

As I mentioned earlier, many people these days seem to be suffering from what Ken Wilber calls new age guilt. They feel that if they get cancer they must have eaten incorrectly or thought the wrong thing or not expressed their emotions properly. That gives them a greater feeling of power than if they say, "I really don't know why I got cancer." There is the sense that what you've created you can uncreate. Of course, for some kinds of cancers this may be true. As a cancer cell biologist, I can tell you that for some cancers in some people, a change in mental factors could change the course of the disease. But there are many other cancers that are biologically determined and couldn't be cured by even the best mental outlook and attitude.

So we need to have a healthy respect for the mystery of things, for the unknown.

Exactly. The Western mind doesn't respect the mystery. It believes that everything is knowable, that if, for example, we were to look hard enough at a particular case of cancer, we would be able to detect every factor that caused it.

In human beings, it seems that the experience of not getting sufficient love as a child, if it doesn't turn into a failure-to-thrive syndrome and death, might in fact turn into shame, into an inherent sense of unworthiness, even if the child wasn't overtly shamed.

That's exactly right. And with that inherent sense of unworthiness, we are prone both to unhealthy guilt and to dealing with healthy guilt in an unhealthy way. When people with a shame-based identity do something wrong, they become so ashamed, so afraid that this really does mean they are worthless and that love will be withdrawn, that they have trouble taking responsibility for their actions and integrating their dark side. Such people develop huge shadows, a huge split between their good and bad sides, like the old story of Jekyll and Hyde. The nice side grows nicer while the shadow gets bigger and darker.

Robert Bly puts it well. He says that we arrive from the far reaches of the universe as 360-degree balls of radiance, place ourselves at our parents' feet, and say, "Here I am." And they say, "I didn't want you, I wanted a good little girl or boy." That's where the drama begins. All the parts of ourselves that are not affirmed or loved get tucked away in the shadow, which he calls a long bag we drag behind us. What we don't see composts in the bag, gets wild, builds up a big head of steam, while we expend all our energy maintaining a mask through which we purchase love and affection. At the same time, we project our dark side onto others. We don't see our own anger, we see the people around us as being angry. We don't see our own sadness, we find sad people to comfort. Unless we begin to heal that split, there's no way we can feel an authentic sense of happiness. When our identity is based on shame, when we have this tremendous fear that unless we are perfect in some way we are not going to be loved, our whole life becomes organized around the avoidance of fear rather than around the attraction of love. The question is, How can we heal this split?

This is the dimension that was missing in your earlier book. There you advised people to meditate and do yoga and perhaps even try psychotherapy, but you didn't address the healing of the split between the true and false selves.

Right. You can do therapy or meditation with the false self and never even touch the authentic self. This authentic self is the repository of all our creativity as well as our full range of emotions, the kinds of emotions that children express so freely, like joy and rage and hurt. When the true self is contacted, these emotions are expressed.

Which is the kind of recognition that tends to accompany the experience of one's authentic self.

Yes. William James understood the problem of pessimism, which he called soul sickness, and the role of shame and guilt and the syndrome of the shame-based personality. The opposite, he said, is healthy-mindedness, and the way to get it is through a true spiritual conversion that affects the very depth of our being and restructures our psychological view of ourselves. And I don't think such a conversion is so hard for people to have.

Why?

The great Indian sage Sri Ramakrishna said, "The winds of grace are blowing all the time, you have only to raise your sail." Jesus said it differently: "Knock and the door will be opened." I see it all the time. We don't get help until we ask. But it's a hard lesson to learn for those of us with a shame-based identity. We don't want to ask for help because we are afraid we'll offend someone or be rejected. We have to learn to ask for help, both psychologically and spiritually. When we truly begin to open ourselves up with an appreciation of the power of nonlocal consciousness and simply say, "May the means for my healing manifest themselves," I believe absolutely that help will be forthcoming. People who put out that message from the depths of their being are usually motivated to follow through and do something that quickens their inner life. Some meditate, some pray, some keep a dream journal, some simply set aside quiet time to invite a bit of sacred silence into their lives. As soon as we begin to open ourselves up, the universe rushes in.

Another thing to remember is that there is power in a group. Being with other people and telling your story can be very healing. In a 12-step program, for example, you realize that you are not the only sinner in the world, and you are not the only one who experiences such terrible guilt and shame. In my experience, people with problems of shame or abuse in childhood who join a 12-step program seem to undergo greater healing than those who just do psychotherapy.

People who belong to meditation or prayer groups report that when they're meditating or praying for someone else, the healing they feel within themselves is remarkable. There is a tremendous sense of love that opens the heart, and suddenly no one has to tell them they are worthy, they know it because they feel it as a flow of love deep inside. Until we feel this flow of love within, we can do all the psychotherapy in the world, and it will just be words.

Resources

Books

Borysenko, J. *Guilt Is the Teacher, Love Is the Lesson*. New York: Warner, 1990.

————. *Minding the Body, Mending the Mind*. New York: Bantam, 1987.

Dossey, L. *Recovery of the Soul*. New York: Bantam, 1991.

Seligman, M. *Helplessness: On Depression, Development and Death*. New York: Freeman, 1975.

————. *Learned Optimism*. New York: Knopf, 1991.

Organizations

Mind/Body Health Sciences, 22 Lawson Terrace, Scituate, MA 02066 (617) 545-7122. Joan Borysenko and her husband, Myrin, offer lectures, workshops, consultations, and trainings for business, hospitals, and other organizations. Also available is an eight-tape set based on the book *Guilt Is the Teacher, Love Is the Lesson*.

Notes

[1] M. Csikszentmihalyi, *Flow: The Psychology of Optimal Experience* (New York, Harper & Row, 1990), p. 6.

[2] Barbara Brown, as quoted in D. E. Davis, A. Eshelman, and M. McKay, *The Relaxation and Stress Reduction Workbook* (Richmond, CA: New Harbinger, 1977), p. 164.

[3] P. Nuernberger, *Freedom from Stress: A Holistic Approach* (Honesdale, PA: Himalayan Institute, 1981), p. 220.

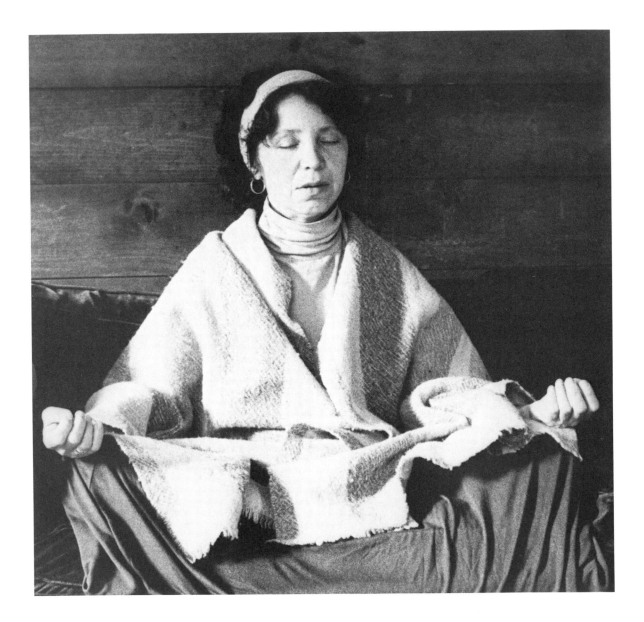

SEVEN

Tapping the Mind's Potential

Relaxation is a stepping-stone toward meditation, and meditation is the royal path to Self-realization, or God consciousness. Meditation is at the very heart of yoga. This chapter introduces you to both the Hindu and Buddhist approaches to meditation. It also explains the connection between the peaceful meditative state and the transcendence of the ego. The down-to-earth advice given in the following essays and interviews will enable you to begin to practice meditation on your own and to encounter the huge potential of your own mind and psyche.

THE NATURE OF THE HUMAN MIND

Philosopher Henryk Skolimowski writes: "Of all the gifts of evolution, mind is the most precious. Yet we have allowed it to become something else than it deserves. Look how much pollution is poured into your mind daily. . . . This garbage in your mind has trivialized your existence, is the cause of anxieties, is the cause of confusion that does not allow you to think right and act appropriately."[1]

These passionate words faithfully mirror the truth proclaimed in the spiritual traditions of the world. The human mind can be either a dumping ground or a treasure trove. We can use our intelligence to create or to destroy, to ennoble our existence or to demean it, to liberate ourselves from the cage of egotism or to chain ourselves to an unworthy fate, to fulfill our highest potential or to live without strength and faith.

Yogis realized long ago that the mind is the alchemical cauldron in which base metal is transmuted into precious gold. It is through

Of all the wonders and mysteries of our universe, nothing is so wondrous as mind.

RAMMURTI S. MISHRA

135

What is mind? It doesn't matter. What is matter? Never mind.

ANONYMOUS

Yoga is without doubt the master key that unlocks the frontiers of the mind.

B. K. S. IYENGAR

the mind, through our own purified or disciplined consciousness, that we can discover our immortal substance, our true identity—the ego-transcending Self (atman). Yoga is the alchemy of transforming our ordinary personality, which is governed by the ego, into an illumined personality that serves the higher purposes of evolution rather than our individual, self-centered desires and schemes. Or more precisely, the intentions of our transmuted personality are in flawless consonance with the larger evolutionary pattern, so that we experience no conflict between what we feel we ought to want and what we actually want.

Those who are heavily invested in their sense of individuality and personal ego's designs find it difficult to understand this state of ego-transcendence. Indeed, they feel threatened by it. Yet, to those who look deeper into life, it is quite obvious that the ego is a psychological function that is given far more credence and prominence than it deserves or is wholesome for us. R. D. Laing, who was one of the most far-seeing psychiatrists of our time, made these pertinent remarks: "True sanity entails in one way or another the dissolution of the normal ego, that false self competently adjusted to our alienated social reality; the emergence of the 'inner' archetypal mediators of divine power, and through this death a rebirth, and the eventual re-establishment of a new kind of ego-functioning, the ego now being the servant of the divine, no longer its betrayer."[2]

Yoga is not a matter of suppressing the ego, or anything else for that matter, but of *transcending* it. We are asked to focus our attention on the "higher" reality, the Self (or God), in which the ego makes its playful appearance. As we discover and recover our true identity, the ego will simply become transparent.

Meditation is the principal yogic means by which we can polish the mind's mirror so that it may reflect the light of the Self without undue distortion. When the mind's blemishes are removed, when we are inwardly balanced and serene, we encounter our true nature. In Zen Buddhist terms, our purified mind reveals itself to be Original Mind. In Hindu terms, pacification of the mental whirls leads to the state of supreme ecstasy in which the transpersonal Self, the Witness, shines forth in its pure state. There is wholeness, fulfillment, and unutterable bliss.

RESOURCES

Books

Arya, U. *Superconscious Meditation*. Honesdale, PA: International Himalayan Institute, 1978.

Brunton, P. *Meditation.* Vol. 4, pt. 1 of *The Notebooks of Paul Brunton.* Burdett, NY: Larson Publications, 1986.

Easwaran, E. *Meditation: A Simple Eight-Point Program for Translating Spiritual Ideals into Daily Life.* Tomales, CA: Nilgiri Press, 2nd ed., 1991.

Feuerstein, G. *Sacred Paths: Essays on Wisdom, Love, and Mystical Realization.* Burdett, NY: Larson Publications, 1991. An information-rich, user-friendly introduction to the principal ideas of yoga.

————. *Wholeness or Transcendence? Ancient Lessons for the Emerging Global Civilization.* Burdett, NY: Larson Publications, 1992. The evolution of the yoga tradition viewed from the perspective of the history of consciousness.

Goleman, D. *The Meditative Mind: The Varieties of Meditative Experience.* Los Angeles: J. P. Tarcher, 1986.

Naranjo, C. *How to Be: Meditation in Spirit and Practice.* Los Angeles: J. P. Tarcher, 1990.

Man is the animal that uses language, responds to beauty, laughs, sheds tears . . . and meditates.

PATRICIA CARRINGTON

THE ROYAL PATH OF MENTAL DISCIPLINE
BY SWAMI VIVEKANANDA

The powers of the mind should be concentrated and turned back upon it; and as the darkest places reveal their secrets before the penetrating rays of the sun, so will the concentrated mind penetrate into its own innermost secrets. Thus shall we come to the basis of belief, the real religion. We shall perceive for ourselves whether or not we have souls, whether or not life lasts for five minutes or for eternity, whether or not there is a God. All this will be revealed to us.

This is what raja yoga proposes to teach. The goal of all its teaching is to show how to concentrate the mind; then how to discover the innermost recesses of our own minds; then how to generalize their contents and form our own conclusions from them. It never asks what our belief is—whether we are deists, or atheists, whether Christians, Jews, or Buddhists. We are human beings, and that is sufficient. Every human being has the right and the power to seek religion; every human being has the right to ask the reason why and to have his question answered by himself—if he only takes the trouble. . . .

The yogi teaches that the mind itself has a higher state of existence, beyond reason, a superconscious state, and that when the mind rises to that state, then this knowledge, which is beyond reason, comes—metaphysical and transcendental knowledge comes to that man. This

137

state of going beyond reason, beyond ordinary human knowledge, may sometimes come by chance to a man who does not understand its science; he stumbles upon it, as it were. When he stumbles upon it, he generally interprets it as coming from outside. So this explains why an inspiration, or transcendental knowledge, may be the same in different countries, but in one country it will seem to come through an angel, and in another through a deva, and in a third through God. What does it mean? It means that the mind brought out the knowledge from within itself and that the manner of finding it was interpreted according to the beliefs and education of the person through whom it came. . . .

All the different steps in yoga are intended to bring us scientifically to the superconscious state, or samadhi. . . . This meditative state is the highest state of existence. So long as there is desire, no real happiness can come. It is only the contemplative, witness-like study of objects that brings us real enjoyment and happiness.

A quiet mind and a quiet vital are the first conditions for success in sadhana [spiritual discipline].

SRI AUROBINDO

THE BUDDHIST YOGA OF MINDFULNESS:
AN INTERVIEW WITH S. N. GOENKA
BY STEPHAN BODIAN

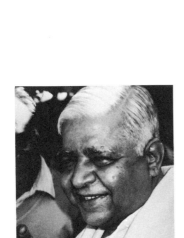

S. N. GOENKA

Next to the Dalai Lama, S. N. Goenka may be the Asian Buddhist teacher best known in the West. His periodic visits to the United States attract large numbers of students, and hundreds flock each year from all parts of the world to attend his ten-day or one-month meditation courses near Bombay.

Although Goenka, born a Hindu, claims to teach the Buddha's original teaching, he does not call himself a Buddhist. "The Dhamma is universal and non-sectarian," he insists. True to this ecumenical orientation, he has taught meditation in Buddhist retreat centers, Hindu temples, and Christian churches, as well as in a Muslim mosque.

Goenka is a master of *vipassana*, popularly known as "insight meditation." He learned this technique from the great Burmese master U Ba Khin, with whom he studied for fourteen years.

What are the techniques of vipassana meditation, as you teach it?

The technique of vipassana is to observe the truth of suffering within oneself, how one becomes agitated, irritated, miserable. One has to go deep within oneself to observe it objectively. Otherwise, the cause of misery always appears to be outside. Say, for example, that I'm angry, and I want to investigate this anger. Even if I close my eyes and try to understand it, the apparent external cause of the anger will keep coming to mind, and I will keep justifying my behavior. "So and so abused me, so and so insulted me, and that's why I am angry. It's no fault of mine." But the fact is, I am miserable.

The technique of vipassana teaches you just to observe. If you are miserable, just observe misery as misery. As you start observing, the cause of misery becomes clear. Because you reacted with negativity, with craving or aversion, you are now experiencing a very unpleasant sensation in the body. But as you keep observing that sensation, it loses its strength and passes away, and the negativity passes with it.

We start with respiration because the mind doesn't become concentrated unless it has an object to focus on. For the first three days of retreat, we observe the breath coming and going at the entrance of the nostrils. As the mind calms down a bit, we start experiencing the sensations around the nostrils and then expand to experience the sensations throughout the body. These sensations take us to the root of our minds. They take us to the root of the misery, to the root of the cause of the misery, and they help us to eradicate that cause. This is what is taught in vipassana.

If I'm not mistaken, the technique of observing the sensations throughout the body is called "sweeping."

Yes, sweeping in the sense that, at a certain stage, all the solidity of the body dissolves. The apparent truth of the material body is solidity. We feel a solid body. But, as you keep observing it objectively, this solidity starts dissolving, and you start experiencing that the entire material structure is nothing but a mass of sub-atomic particles arising and passing away, arising and passing away. The entire body is just a mass of vibration.

At first, however, when you are still with the solidity, you can't sweep, can't get a flow of vibration throughout the body, because there are blockages here and there—pain, pressure, heaviness. Instead, you keep observing part by part, and little by little all that solidity dissolves, and you reach the stage of total dissolution, mere vibration. Then your attention can move easily from the head to the feet and back again without any obstruction. This is what I refer to as "sweeping."

So sweeping occurs when you are totally clear.

If you leave your mind as it is, it will become calm. This mind is called big mind.

SHUNRYU SUZUKI

Real meditation is not purposive. It has no effect that it seeks to produce. It has no dilemma to solve.

DA FREE JOHN
(LOVE-ANANDA)

139

You are a system of Light, as are all beings. The frequency of your Light depends upon your consciousness. When you shift the level of your consciousness, you shift the frequency of your Light.

GARY ZUKAV

Totally—when there is no blockage anywhere. The Buddha says: "By this technique, a student learns how to feel the entire body in one breath. Breathing in, you feel the entire body. Breathing out, you feel the entire body." This happens only when the body dissolves, when all solidity disappears. Then as you breathe out, you feel from head to feet; as you breathe in, you feel from feet to head. That is what we call sweeping—a stage where the body dissolves and intense mental contents dissolve as well. If there are strong emotions, you can't get this sweeping, because strong emotions result in a feeling of solidity in the body. When emotions are dissolved at the mental level, and the solidity of the body is dissolved at the material level, nothing remains but a mass of vibration, a mass of energy moving in the body.

Ideally, one would be able to do this all the time, throughout the day.

Yes. Once one reaches this stage, one continues to work with sweeping. But certain conditionings or impurities of the past, called *sankharas* [*samskaras* in Sanskrit], may exist at a very deep level of the mind. Through this sweeping, moving from head to feet and feet to head, these impurities get shaken and start coming to the surface. Say a certain sankhara manifests itself as gross sensations in the body. You work on these gross sensations by just observing them, until they too dissolve and you again get a free flow.

The goal of this technique is not to achieve the free flow of vibrations, which is after all just another transitory experience, but to accept with equanimity whatever manifests itself. In this way, you eradicate your mental conditioning layer by layer, and along with it your suffering.

RESOURCES

Books

Fields, R. *How the Swans Came to the Lake: A Narrative History of Buddhism in America*. Boston, MA: Shambhala, 1986.

Goldstein, J. *The Experience of Insight: A Natural Unfolding*. Boston, MA: Shambhala, 1987.

Hart, H. *The Art of Living: Vipassana Meditation as Taught by S. N. Goenka*. San Francisco: Harper & Row, 1987.

Kornfield, J. *Living Buddhist Masters*. Santa Cruz, CA: Unity Press, 1977.

Organizations

Insight Meditation Society, Pleasant Street, Barre, MA 01005. Tel. (508) 355-4378.

Insight Meditation West, 5000 Sir Francis Drake Boulevard, Woodacre, CA 94973. Tel. (415) 488-0164.

Vipassana Meditation Center, P.O. Box 24, Shelburne Falls, MA 01370. Tel. (413) 625-2160. This is S. N. Goenka's center in the United States.

SUFFERING IS NOT ENOUGH
BY THICH NHAT HANH

Life is filled with suffering, but it is also filled with many wonders, like the blue sky, the sunshine, the eyes of a baby. To suffer is not enough. We must also be in touch with the wonders of life. They are within us and all around us, everywhere, any time.

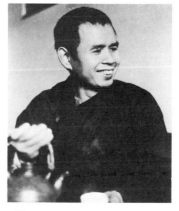

THICH NHAT HANH

If we are not happy, if we are not peaceful, we cannot share peace and happiness with others, even those we love, those who live under the same roof. If we are peaceful, if we are happy, we can smile and blossom like a flower, and everyone in our family, our entire society, will benefit from our peace. Do we need to make a special effort to enjoy the beauty of the blue sky? Do we have to practice to be able to enjoy it? No, we just enjoy it. Each second, each minute of our lives can be like this. Wherever we are, any time, we have the capacity to enjoy the sunshine, the presence of each other, even the sensation of our breathing. We don't need to go to China to enjoy the blue sky. We don't have to travel into the future to enjoy our breathing. We can be in touch with these things right now. It would be a pity if we were only aware of suffering.

We are so busy we hardly have time to look at the people we love, even in our own household, and to look at ourselves. Society is organized in a way that even when we have some leisure time, we don't know how to use it to get back in touch with ourselves. We have millions of ways to lose this precious time—we turn on the TV or pick up the telephone, or start the car and go somewhere. We are not used to being with ourselves, and we act as if we don't like ourselves and are trying to escape from ourselves.

Meditation is to be aware of what is going on—in our bodies, in our feelings, in our minds, and in the world. Each day 40,000 children die of hunger. The superpowers now have more than 50,000 nuclear warheads, enough to destroy our planet many times. Yet the sunrise is beautiful, and the rose that bloomed this morning along the wall is a miracle. Life is both dreadful and wonderful. To practice meditation is to be in touch with both aspects. Please do not think we must be solemn in order to meditate. In fact, to meditate well, we have to smile a lot.

From time to time, to remind ourselves to relax, to be peaceful, we may wish to set aside some time for a retreat, a day of mindfulness, when we can walk slowly, smile, drink tea with a friend, enjoy being together as if we were the happiest people on Earth. This is not a retreat, it is a treat. During walking meditation, during kitchen and garden work, during sitting meditation, all day long, we can practice smiling. At first you may find it difficult to smile, and we have to think about why. Smiling means that we are ourselves, that we have sovereignty over ourselves, that we are not drowned into forgetfulness. This kind of smile can be seen on the faces of Buddhas and bodhisattvas.

Even though life is hard, even though it is sometimes difficult to smile, we have to try. Just as when we wish each other, "Good morning," it must be a real "Good morning." Recently, one friend asked me, "How can I force myself to smile when I am filled with sorrow? It isn't natural." I told her she must be able to smile to her sorrow, because we are more than our sorrow. A human being is like a television set with millions of channels. If we turn the Buddha on, we are the Buddha. If we turn sorrow on, we are sorrow. If we turn a smile on, we really are the smile. We cannot let just one channel dominate us. We have the seed of everything in us, and we have to seize the situation in our hand, to recover our own sovereignty.

When we sit down peacefully, breathing and smiling, with awareness, we are our true selves, we have sovereignty over ourselves. When we open ourselves up to a TV program, we let ourselves be invaded by the program. Sometimes it is a good program, but often it is just noisy. Because we want to have something other than ourselves enter us, we sit there and let a noisy television program invade us, assail us, destroy us. Even if our nervous system suffers, we don't have the courage to stand up and turn it off, because if we do that, we will have to return to our self.

Meditation is the opposite. It helps us return to our true self. Practicing meditation in this kind of society is very difficult. Everything seems to work in concert to try to take us away from our true self. We have thousands of things, like video tapes and music, which help us be away from ourselves. Practicing meditation is to be aware, to smile, to

In the beginning, meditation proves very difficult and dry. But if you persist, as in the taking of a medicine, you will find in it a perennial source of joy, pure and unalloyed.

SWAMI BRAHMANANDA

breathe. These are on the opposite side. We go back to ourselves in order to see what is going on, because to meditate means to be aware of what is going on. What is going on is very important. . . .

If we are not able to smile, then the world will not have peace. It is not by going out for a demonstration against nuclear missiles that we can bring about peace. It is with our capacity of smiling, breathing, and being peace that we can make peace.

RESOURCES

Books

Thich Nhat Hanh. *Zen Poems.* Greensboro, NC: Unicorn, 1976.

————. *A Guide to Walking Meditation.* Nyack, NY: Fellowship of Reconciliation, 1985.

————. *Being Peace.* Berkeley, CA: Parallax Press, 1987.

————. *Old Path, White Clouds.* Berkeley, CA: Parallax Press, 1991.

————. *Peace Is Every Step.* New York: Bantam, 1991.

Further works by Thich Nhat Hanh are available from Parallax Press, P. O. Box 7355, Berkeley, CA 94707. Tel. (510) 525-0101.

Organizations

Community of Mindful Living, a nonprofit organization founded by Thich Nhat Hanh in 1991, is dedicated to relief work in Vietnam and to promoting the founder's teaching. The address is the same as Parallax Press.

Fellowship of Reconciliation, founded in 1916, is an international organization dedicated to nonviolent social change and the promotion of peace and justice in the world through creative and compassionate reconciliation. The address is: 523 North Broadway, Nyack, NY 10960-0271. Tel. (914) 358-4601.

THE EGO AND MEDITATION
BY RAM DASS

The ego has convinced us that we need it—not only that we need it, but that we are it. I am my body. I am my personality. I am my neuroses. I am angry. I am depressed.

> *There is only one level of consciousness that cannot accept the universal on-off switch, and that is the ego.*
>
> TIMOTHY LEARY

143

I'm a good person. I'm sincere. I seek truth. I'm a lazy slob. Definition after definition. Room after room. Some are in high-rise apartments—I'm very important. Some are on the fringe of the city—just hanging out.

Meditation raises the question: Who are we really? If we are the same as our ego, then if we open up the ego's filters and overwhelm it, we shall be drowned. If, on the other hand, we are not exclusively what the ego defines us to be, then the removal of the ego's filters may not be such a great threat. It may actually mean our liberation. But as long as the ego calls the shots, we can never become other than what it says. Like a dictator, it offers us paternalistic security at the expense of our freedom.

We may ask how we could survive without our ego. Don't worry—it doesn't disappear. We can learn to venture beyond it, though. The ego is there, as our servant. Our room is there. We can always go in and use it like an office when we need to be efficient. But the door can be left open so that we can always walk out.

THE POWER AND LIMITS OF MEDITATION
BY KEN WILBER

Meditation is not a way to make things easier; it's a way to make them worse, so you will have to grow in the process.

The worst pitfall, I would say, is using meditation to "spiritually bypass" other concerns, concerns that can only be handled in their own terms, or on their own level. People think that meditation will take care of their money problems, their sex problems, their food problems—and of course it won't. What it will do is make you more sensitive and aware; and if you've got a painful life problem, meditation will probably just make it more painful because it will make you more sensitive. Meditation means you can't hide the pain anymore. You have to step right into the middle of it.

In particular, meditation will not take care of most psychological problems. If you're basically a neurotic, meditation will make you a nice, enlightened neurotic. If you're a real schmuck, meditation will make you a real sensitive schmuck. It doesn't eliminate fundamental psychological or neurotic difficulties, and in some cases it can make them worse.

Are you saying that meditation is of no use at all with psychological problems?

No, no, I wouldn't say that. It can be of benefit in many ways, particularly in strengthening witnessing-awareness, but preferably along-

The mind is a camera: it creates, perceives, and records reality. Its depth is unfathomable; its breadth unimaginable; its energy boundless.

GABRIELLE ROTH

side a psychotherapy designed to deal specifically and directly with your particular neurosis. My point is that many people think that meditation is some sort of panacea, and it isn't. It is a direct way to engage your own growth and evolution, and, as is always the case, growth is painful. It hurts. If you're doing meditation correctly, you are in for some very rough and frightening times. Meditation as a "relaxation response" is a joke. Genuine meditation involves a whole series of deaths and rebirths; extraordinary conflicts and stresses come into play. All of this is just barely balanced by an equal growth in equanimity, compassion, understanding, awareness, and sensitivity, which makes the whole endeavor worthwhile.

But it's not just a day at the beach. Look at the life stories of the great saints and sages, and you will see tremendous struggle and pain. And notice that most of it starts after they have progressed in meditation, not before. My point is that there are extraordinary benefits and extraordinary pains, so hang in there. Just don't meditate instead of taking out the garbage—physical, emotional, or psychological.

Practice is absolutely necessary.

SWAMI VIVEKANANDA

TIPS FOR MEDITATION

1. It is possible to meditate at any time, but an ideal time is at sunrise.

2. It promotes your inner work to practice regularly and at least once, ideally twice, a day (morning and evening).

3. Never force yourself to meditate. There should be something of a joyous anticipation about sitting in meditation.

4. Take advantage of those moments when you feel naturally meditative.

5. Quiet surroundings are obviously helpful to the meditative process. Outer harmony (such as found in a beautiful park or at a picturesque lake) furthers inner balance. At home, it is helpful to create a special place for meditation. Ask your family to cooperate with you by not disturbing your meditation.

6. Prepare for your meditation session by washing your hands and face, and generally freshening up. This dispels drowsiness and promotes a wakeful, energetic disposition.

7. It is good to sit with the spine straight, whether it be on a chair or on the floor in the lotus posture.

8. Begin by taking a few deep breaths, expelling all tensions in the body and concerns of the mind.

9. Consciously relax your entire body, especially the chest and the facial muscles.

10. Resolve to dedicate yourself to the meditation process whole-heartedly.

11. Tell yourself, mentally or aloud, that for the duration of the meditation nothing else matters.

12. Be willing to surrender your self and encounter the greater Being.

13. If this is meaningful to you, remember the joy you felt when you last contacted your innermost essence. Alternatively, re-call incidents of happiness in your life, which expanded your sense of being present in the body.

14. Now begin your meditation practice, whatever your tech-nique may be: the practice of mindfulness, mantra recitation, contemplation of a particularly meaningful image, or abstract concentration.

15. Don't be concerned about distracting thoughts, sensations, and emotions. Neither welcome them nor repress them. Sim-ply persist in your practice. Sooner or later your inner world will become calm.

16. There are no "good" or "bad" meditations. All that matters is that you seriously engage the meditative process, regardless of the content that arises. Every meditation is a step toward greater inner freedom.

17. Don't abandon your meditation at the first impulse to do so, especially when the going is rough. Stick with it for a while. Try to sit for at least fifteen minutes at the beginning, and af-ter a few weeks of practice, for at least half an hour. Often you can overcome the initial resistance, and then you may find yourself in a completely different inner space. You will learn to recognize that there is a natural ending to every medita-tion, where it seems appropriate to get up.

18. After your meditation is over, review the session and affirm its positive aspects.

19. Throughout the day, try to recall the inner peace created by deep meditation.

20. Don't overmeditate. If you wish to meditate for several hours a day, it would be wise to do so under the supervision of a qualified teacher.

21. Take on the discipline of not chatting about your meditation experiences to everyone, which would merely dissipate your psychic energy.

Notes

[1] H. Skolimowsky, *Ecological Renaissance* (Ann Arbor, MI: Eco-Philosophy Centre, 1991), p. 5.

[2] R. D. Laing, *The Politics of Experience* (New York: Pantheon, 1967), p. 145.

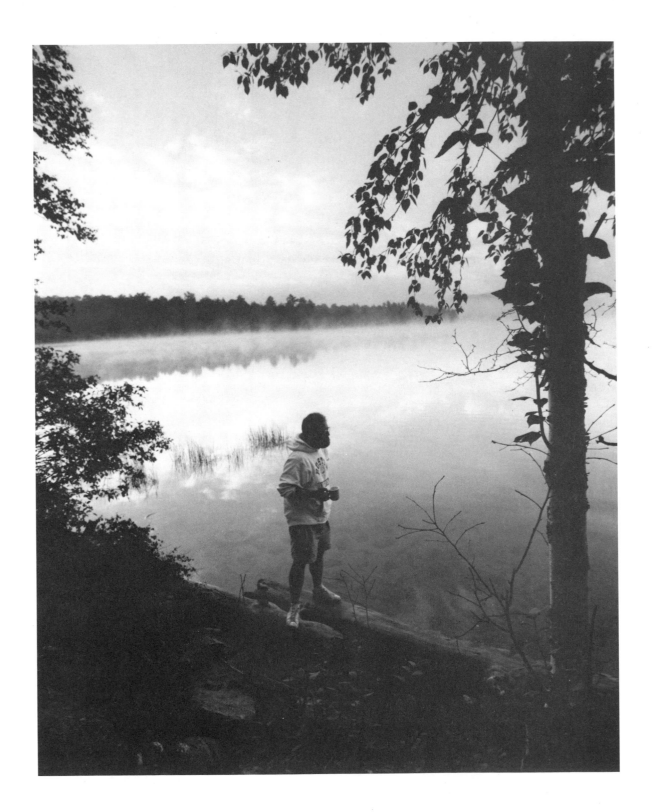

EIGHT

Expanding Awareness

Meditation is like a sixth sense. It leads to an expanded awareness, opening up new horizons for experiencing reality. This chapter explores some of the unconventional areas associated with meditation and higher yogic practice. You will read about how psychologists look upon the extraordinary states of consciousness to which regular yoga practice provides access. You will also learn about possible dangers on the path of meditation, including hypersensitivity.

Finally, since meditation is best learned from a qualified teacher, the question of how to relate to spiritual teachers is addressed at some length. Yoga has from the beginning been an initiatory path, and many contemporary schools of yoga follow a similar structure: a teacher, who is usually charismatic, imparts esoteric knowledge and "transmits" spiritual experiences to a disciple. Thus, a teacher, or guru, is invested with considerable authority over his or her disciples. In recent years, the mass media have exposed many cases of questionable and even immoral and unlawful behavior on the part of spiritual teachers.

How can you prevent disappointment and protect yourself against abuse? How can you benefit from a teacher-disciple relationship without running the risk of disempowering yourself and stunting your personal growth? This chapter provides sound and helpful answers.

WALKING ON THE RAZOR'S EDGE

Even though we are never really separated from our true nature, the Self, we nonetheless feel separated from it. This is in fact the malaise of our egoic existence. Rediscovery of our true identity is sudden, but it is

Our self-membranes should not be too tightly sealed, because we require constant inflow from the Ground to renew and sustain our vitality. The infinitely abundant Ground is our life force.

JOHN E. NELSON

typically preceded by a long and arduous process of removing one obstruction after another. In the course of that purifying process, we progressively discover the hidden aspects of the mind and psyche and, ultimately, the Self (atman or purusha) itself.

As we tread the path to Self-realization, we become naturally more sensitive. At times this can prove to be its own obstacle, because we may find it difficult to deal with the onslaught of information that enters our highly sensitized psyche. We also may acquire unusual psychic abilities, which are known as *siddhis* in yoga.

Our further spiritual growth depends largely on how we relate to all these new possibilities that spring to life within us. If we exploit them for selfish ends, we are apt to lose sight of our spiritual aspiration altogether and then bring great harm upon ourselves and possibly others. This is why yoga insists on a firm moral foundation. The spiritual path has been compared to a razor's edge, and the only way in which we can avoid cutting ourselves is by cultivating absolute integrity.

All too often one hears of teachers who seem to behave in ways that are morally doubtful or reprehensible. Paranormal abilities and personal magnetism or charisma are no sure guarantee that a person is spiritually mature. While we can benefit greatly from teachers who are genuine and competent, we also can be hurt by impostors and those who have donned the teacher's mantle prematurely.

Hence we must exercise caution and discrimination in our choice of teachers, just as we must be constantly vigilant about our own actions and motives. Yoga is grounded in discernment (viveka) between truth and falsehood, reality and illusion. So long as we keep our gaze firmly fixed on the highest possible ideals, deception and self-deception can find no anchorage in our lives. In this way, we shall continue to walk and grow in the light.

To change your mind is to change your body, to function differently.

STANLEY KELEMAN

BEYOND EGO
BY BRYAN WITTINE, PH.D.

The Ageless Wisdom of Transpersonal Psychology

There is a famous Sufi story found in Idries Shah's *Tales of the Dervishes* in which a young prince is told by his parents that he must journey from his homeland to alien shores, and there find a precious jewel guarded by a monster. In doing so, he is to achieve a degree of awareness and enlightenment that cannot be attained except by making this journey.

After providing him with a special food to sustain him during his exile, the king and queen send their son on his way. But once he arrives at his destination, he falls into a kind of trance that affects just about everyone in this strange, dreamlike land. Donning the garb of the country and engaging in an occupation befitting a good citizen, he forgets his true home and mission.

Learning of his distress, the people of the prince's native land send him a message: "Awake! For you are the son of royal parents. You were sent on a special mission and to us you must return."

The message awakens the prince. He finds the monster, uses special sounds to put it to sleep, and seizes the priceless jewel. Then, using the same sounds, he retraces his steps back to his native land.

There are many versions of this story, whose central figure is the human spirit traveling on a path to fulfill his or her destiny and return to his or her true home—from the *Odyssey*, to the story of the prodigal son, to "The Hymn of the Soul" in *The Acts of Thomas* in the Aprocryphal New Testamant. While traveling in Asia, one acquaintance said he saw this same story performed as a ritualistic dance in a huge cave.

This story lies at the heart of transpersonal psychology, a modern expression of the world's ageless wisdom. According to Aldous Huxley, this wisdom, known as the perennial philosophy, is "the metaphysic that recognizes a divine Reality substantial to the world of things and lives and minds; the psychology that finds in the soul something similar to, or even identical with, divine Reality; the ethic that places man's final end in the knowledge of the immanent and transcendent Ground of all being."[1] More specifically, Huxley was referring to an esoteric tradition that he believed is at the core of Hinduism, Buddhism, Taoism, Sufism, and Christian mysticism.

As a modern expression of the ageless wisdom, transpersonal psychology seeks to expand the field of psychological inquiry into the farther reaches of human consciousness. It inquires into the entire journey of the human spirit as symbolized by the king's son: his or her descent into physical form; his or her realization of the jewel of individual selfhood that must be differentiated from the trance of everyday life and the ogre of primitive human emotion; and his or her eventual return to the true Self, to the original unity and wholeness which, paradoxically, he or she never really left.

The esoteric tradition tells us that we come from (or are grounded in) the One Self, that we are estranged from or unaware of our origin, and that we can return not through learning, but by remembering our true identity. Each esoteric form has its own way of saying it. For example, in Christian mysticism we are to marry Christ as the Beloved and

It is hard to read Jung, Eliade or Campbell or Huxley without being permanently affected in our perceptions.

ABRAHAM MASLOW

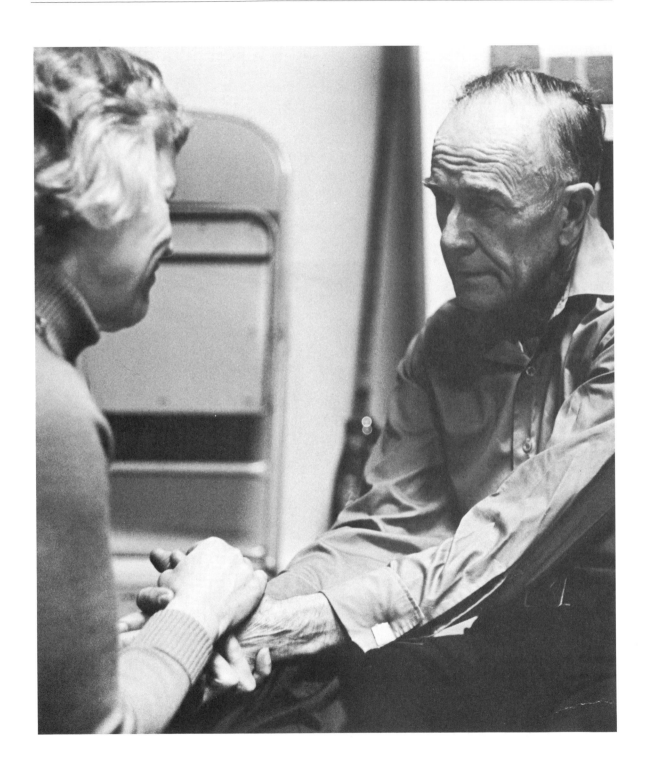

enter the Kingdom of God. Buddhists speak of awakening to our Buddha nature. In the yogas of India, the goal is to realize the Atman. Many transpersonal psychologists speak of realizing the Self, the deep center of Being.

How, we may ask, did a view of the Self from the perennial wisdom become the heart of a psychology? After all, isn't psychology, at least in this country's academic institutions, concerned with rats and objective tests and empirical provability rather than with the feelingful human being? And don't most forms of psychotherapy teach us to adjust, adapt, and strengthen our egos, rather than transcending them? For the most part, this is true. But the roots of the word "psychology" are the Greek *psulche,* meaning "spirit, soul, life, breath," and *logos,* meaning "word, speech, reason." Psychology, then, originally meant the word or language of the spirit or soul.

The word "transpersonal" (from the Latin *trans,* meaning "beyond, through," and *persona,* meaning "mask"), was adopted to reflect the reports of individuals who were practicing various meditative techniques and experiencing states of consciousness extending beyond the customary ego boundaries and the ordinary limitations of time and space. It also has been defined as referring to the release of transcendental attributes, such as altruistic love and compassion, through the daily activities of the personality. The word also can be seen simply as an amalgam of "transcendental" and "personal." One purpose of transpersonal psychology, then, is to help us integrate the transcendental or spiritual and the personal dimensions of existence, to help us fulfill our unique, creative individuality while pointing toward our rootedness in the deep, non-temporal, formless dimension of eternal Being. Therefore, if psychology was originally the study of the spirit or soul, transpersonal psychology is a throwback to earlier days.

However we define it, transpersonal psychology has a venerable ancestry. Ken Wilber, the most influential and prolific writer in transpersonal psychology today, suggests that the field goes all the way back to Plato, Augustine, and Plotinus in the West, and Patanjali, Buddhaghosha, and Asanga in the East. In this century, its contributors have included William James, C. G. Jung, Roberto Assagioli, and Abraham Maslow, and the field currently offers books and articles by Wilber, Stanislav Grof, Frances Vaughan, Roger Walsh, Ralph Metzner, and John Welwood, among others. These writers have been influenced not only by Eastern and Western esoteric psychologies, but by contemporary scientists like David Bohm, Rupert Sheldrake, Ilya Prigogine, and

The natural history of the mind is no further advanced today than was natural science in the thirteenth century. We have only begun to take scientific note of our spiritual experiences.

C. G. JUNG

others whose views on space, time, matter, energy, life, and consciousness parallel, at least to some extent, the findings of sages and mystics.

The Background of Transpersonal Psychology

Transpersonal psychology had its start in the late 1960s, when encounter groups, psychedelics, flower children, and Vietnam war protests were part of this country's creative ferment. At that time, a "third force"—humanistic psychology—was emerging to counterbalance the reductionistic scientific materialism of behaviorism, the "first force," and Freudian psychoanalysis, the "second force." Behaviorism, with its conditioning experiments on rats and pigeons, and psychoanalysis, founded on Freud's theory of the mind as a complex biological machine, seemed to humanistic psychologists to miss the human being as a person—one who is aware, choiceful, intentional, related to others, and capable of actualizing his or her unique creative potentials.

Within this "third force," several individuals began exploring the relevance of Eastern religions and non-orthodox Western psychologies. In particular, they believed Eastern spirituality, with its emphasis on self-transcendence, could be integrated with the humanistic perspective and its focus on self-actualization. In 1968, Abraham Maslow, author of two classic works on humanistic psychology, *Toward a Psychology of Being* and *The Farther Reaches of Human Nature*, stated, "I consider Humanistic, Third Force Psychology to be transitional, a preparation for a still 'higher' Fourth psychology, transpersonal, transhuman, centered in the cosmos rather than in human needs and interests, going beyond humanness, identity, self-actualization, and the like."[2]

Maslow, who died in 1970, criticized behaviorism for representing human beings as animals conditioned by their environment, and Freud for developing his model of human behavior from the study of mental illness. "Freud supplied to us the sick half of psychology," he wrote, "and we must now fill it out with the healthy half." Without Maslow and his colleague, Anthony Sutich, the founding editor for both the *Journal of Humanistic Psychology* and the *Journal of Transpersonal Psychology*, the new orientation might not have emerged.

The Pioneer Efforts of Jung and Assagioli

Although Maslow and Sutich were primarily responsible for consolidating transpersonal psychology into a distinctive field, there existed at least two earlier Western approaches to the transpersonal. These were the efforts of C. G. Jung, one of Freud's most distinguished pupils, and a relatively unknown Italian psychiatrist, Roberto Assagioli, who

Be very careful about locating good or God, right or wrong, legal or illegal, at your favorite level of consciousness.

TIMOTHY LEARY

Ego-consciousness, let alone the tradition of modern individualism, is a phenomenon with a comparatively short history; it is hardly essential for human survival or for a rich human culture, and may ultimately be inimical to both.

MORRIS BERMAN

founded a system called psychosynthesis. Jungian analysis and psycho-synthesis have become two of the most respected approaches within the growing field of transpersonal psychotherapy.

Jung can be called the first representative of a transpersonal orientation in psychology, for while he placed great emphasis upon the dynamics of the personality, as had Freud, his conceptualization of the deeper strata of the human being went far beyond that of his senior.

For Jung, the unconscious was creative and intelligent, and it connected the individual to humanity, nature, and the cosmos. The personal unconscious, for Jung, was a harbor that opens out onto a great ocean he called the collective unconscious. The personal unconscious is constantly fed by the waters of the collective, which Jung and many of his followers called transpersonal. It exists above and beyond and surrounding the individual psyche, and the individual consciousness grows in its soil. From a careful study of his own and his patients' dreams and fantasies, his numerous world travels, and his penetrating analyses of comparative religion, world mythology, and symbolism, Jung found "collectively present dynamic patterns" formed by the remote experiences of humanity. The contents of this deeper strata are identical in all human beings and are expressed in symbols found in all cultures. These universal themes and leitmotifs were called the archetypes of the collective unconscious. For instance, the king's son is a classic example of the "hero archetype." So is the prince who awakened Sleeping Beauty with a kiss.

At the center of this archetypal realm exists an authority to whom the hero must surrender. Jung called this central figure the Self. His conception of the Self as the "God within us" or the inner deity, a supreme directing force superordinate to the personality, gives Jung his indisputable place in transpersonal psychology.

Contrary to the position of the perennial wisdom, however, Jung believed it is dangerous for the individual ego to dissolve into the Self. He believed the ego and Self needed to become related, but that the greater should never overcome the lesser. "It must be reckoned a catastrophe when the ego is assimilated by the Self," he wrote, for such a dissolution could lead to psychosis. Thus, the king's son can be in relationship to his homeland, symbol of the true Self, but he may never fully return there until after death. In this way, Jung's position is contrary to the principles of the ageless wisdom and the findings of advanced meditation practitioners. Many who persist in the practice of spiritual disciplines can and do dissolve their individual consciousness into the Self, at least temporarily.

The individual mind is immanent but not only in the body. It is immanent also in pathways and messages outside the body; and there is a larger Mind of which the individual mind is only a sub-system. This larger Mind is comparable to God and is perhaps what some people mean by "God," but it is still immanent in the total interconnected social system and planetary ecology.

GREGORY BATESON

All human beings have the ability to know themselves and to think rationally.

HERACLITUS

Roberto Assagioli also disagreed with Jung's position. As early as 1910, he began to formulate a model of growth psychology he came to call psychosynthesis. Assagioli pioneered psychoanalysis in his native Italy but quickly became aware of its limitations. Psychoanalysis, he said, focused exclusively on "the basement of human nature"—our conflicting drives, our sexual repressions, our primitive urges—and tended to reduce authentic spiritual and religious yearnings to neurotic, infantile impulses.

For Assagioli, the task was to examine not only the basement of the human being, but the entire mansion. Psychosynthesis was the second major approach in Western psychology to specifically address the farther reaches of human nature—our creative impulses, our urges toward humanitarian action, love, and beauty, and in particular the possibility of realizing what Assagioli called the higher or spiritual Self. In this work, Assagioli was influenced by a number of spiritual teachings, including Hindu yoga, theosophy, Buddhism, and Christian mysticism.

Like Jung, whose views he greatly admired, Assagioli recognized a distinction between the personal "I," a point of pure self-awareness and ruler of the personality, and the higher Self. However, paradoxically, there is no real dichotomy between them. For Assagioli, there is only one Self, but several distinct levels of Self-realization. In the first, our sense of "I" is experienced as distinct contents of our personalities. In most of us, the "I" is usually confused with our emotions, thoughts, desires, the roles we play, and our various identities. If we disidentify from these changing contents by using special psychosynthesis techniques, we can learn they are not really who we are.

In the second stage of realization, the Self is recognized as a separate entity existing above and beyond the personal self. The mystical poetry of Kabir and St. John of the Cross are excellent expressions of this degree of realization. We participate in a deeper dimension of Being, but preserve at the same time a vivid, even sharpened sense of individual identity.

But the duality between the I and the Self is only an appearance. The Self is no more separate from the I than our palm is separate from our fingers. Consequently, at an even further stage of Self-realization, Assagioli says we transcend the illusion of separateness altogether.

Ken Wilber's Spectrum of Identity

In transpersonal psychology, it was Ken Wilber who finally developed a model encompassing the various levels of identity realized by the king's son in his journey from trance state to return. In *The Spectrum of Consciousness* and *No Boundary*, two early works, Wilber asks us to consider the question "Who am I?" Our answers, he claims, depend entirely upon where we draw the line between what we identify as "I" and what we exclude as "not-I." When I describe myself, I am identified with everything on the inside of that boundary line. Everything not me is outside.

According to Wilber, the Self, unity consciousness, or Mind is the nature and condition of all sentient beings. As a result of our conditioning, however, we limit ourselves and our world and turn from our original nature to embrace a boundaried existence. "Our originally pure consciousness," Wilber wrote, "then functions on various levels, with different identities and different boundaries. These different levels are basically the many ways we can and do answer the question 'Who am I?'"[3]

Where we draw our boundary is arbitrary; it can and frequently does shift. It can also be redrawn. A basic hypothesis of transpersonal psychology is that healing and growth accompany a gradual redrawing of the boundary line to include more of the outer as inner, more of the not-self as self.

According to Wilber, as we redraw the boundary between our body-mind and the unitive state, we may develop various transpersonal qualities (such as love, wisdom, and serenity); various extrasensory faculties (such as intuition, clairvoyance, and telepathy); visions of archetypal figures (the wise old man or woman, an inner Christ or Buddha); revelations of light and sound; and feelings of rapture and bliss. Ultimately, these transpersonal bands culminate in the level of Mind, the realization of a transpersonal Self. We remember our fundamental identity with a formless, non-temporal ground of being which transcends all boundaries and all subject/object distinctions. The Self, we discover, is the essence of the entire world, of all worlds, inner and outer, and of all levels of identity, high and low, above and below.

Returning Home from Exile

Research in transpersonal psychology has shown what spiritual traditions have emphasized for centuries: as we progress on the spiritual path and awaken to the Self, we become, paradoxically, more selfless. As we lessen our concern with our personal dramas and open more fully to the heartbeat of humanity, our individual lives become more dedicated to relieving the suffering of others.

Humanity in our time is "dispirited"—and the results have been

When we awake the self mysteriously re-appears, we do not know how or whence—a fact which, if closely examined, is truly baffling and disturbing. This leads us to assume that the re-appearance of the conscious self or ego is due to the existence of a permanent center, of a true Self situated beyond or "above" it.

ROBERT ASSAGIOLI

disastrous. Our environment is being ravaged, our natural resources are dwindling, and the specter of destruction looms like a giant shadow darkening the future of our planet. This chaos is reflected in today's illnesses of the soul. What human being has not, at one point or another, felt his or her spirit sapped by isolation, meaninglessness, and paralyzing fear?

As I see it, humanity's dispiritedness is the result of being cut off from its roots in eternal Being. Do we not hunger for spiritual food? Are we not, each of us, reaching for a greater unity? Are we not yearning for that supreme synthesis in which our separated selves are at least temporarily nourished by being dissolved in the fullness of the divine?

Life in exile is indeed filled with suffering, as the Buddha so plainly taught. Transpersonal psychology teaches that we cannot remain in exile and survive. Although appearances tell us otherwise, nothing is really separate from the universal Self. We are at a crossroads in our evolutionary journey, a planetary existential crisis. We are being called upon to choose between total annihilation and a radical transformation of who we are, from isolated egos struggling for survival to beings in touch with our essential divinity. We are the king's sons, the king's daughters, and each of us is on the journey home again. Transpersonal psychology is one approach working to speed us on our way.

Fortunately, healthy people experience almost daily flashes of "vision"—the peak experience—which make us aware that there is something badly wrong with our basic assumptions: they bring the flash of "absurd good news."

COLIN WILSON

RESOURCES

Books

Assagioli, R. *Psychosynthesis: A Manual of Principles and Techniques.* New York: Viking Press, 1965. A pioneering work in transpersonal psychology, combining theory and practice.

Hoffman, E. *The Right to Be Human: A Biography of Abraham Maslow.* Los Angeles: J. P. Tarcher, 1988.

Jung, C. G. *Memories, Dreams and Reflections.* New York: Vintage, 1965.

Maslow, A. *The Farther Reaches of Human Nature.* New York: Viking, 1971. A groundbreaking work, which can still be read with profit.

Wilber, K. *The Atman Project: A Transpersonal View of Human Development.* Wheaton, IL.: Quest Books, 1980.

_____. *The Spectrum of Consciousness.* Wheaton, IL: Quest Books, 1977. Wilber's first and best known book, which is a remarkable synthesis of Eastern and Western ideas on the human psyche.

Periodicals

Journal of Humanistic Psychology, published quarterly by Sage Publications, 2455 Teller Road, Newbury Park, CA 91320.

Journal of Transpersonal Psychology, published biannually by the Association for Transpersonal Psychology, P.O. Box 4437, Stanford, CA 94305.

ReVision, published quarterly by Heldref Publications, 4000 Albemarle Street, NW, Washington, DC 20016.

Organizations

Association for Humanistic Psychology, 1772 Vallejo Street #3, San Francisco, CA 94123. The Association publishes the *Journal of Humanistic Psychology* and organizes conferences. Tel. (415) 346-7929.

Association for Transpersonal Psychology is a branch of the Transpersonal Institute, a nonprofit organization located at 345 California Avenue #1, Palo Alto, CA 94306. Tel. (415) 327-2066.

COMMON GROUND BETWEEN PSYCHOTHERAPY AND SPIRITUALITY
BY FRANCES VAUGHAN, PH.D.

1. **Telling the truth.** Communicating the truth about inner experience is essential for effective change and growth. Psychotherapy provides a safe space for this.

2. **Releasing negative emotions.** Letting go of fear, guilt, and anger can be facilitated by therapeutic interventions, and is valuable for both personal and spiritual work.

3. **Effort and consistency.** Progress in personal and spiritual development can be enhanced by effort and consistency, although too much effort may be counterproductive. Understanding resistance in psychotherapy can be valuable for anyone exploring spiritual growth. The ability to make a consistent effort, to follow through on intentions, and to behave in a way that is consistent with professed beliefs are fundamental requirements for all inner work.

4. **Authenticity and trust.** Authenticity is strengthened when what one says and does accurately reflects what one thinks and feels. It is necessary if one is to avoid self-deception and develop self-trust. When

people feel untrustworthy, they cannot trust their perceptions of others or the world. Self-trust is necessary even in choosing a therapist or a teacher.

5. Integrity and wholeness. Integrity results from the practice of authenticity, and wholeness depends on accepting all one's experience. Allowing things to be as they are rather than living in a world of illusion and denial is basic for psychological health and spiritual growth.

6. Insight and forgiveness. To understand all is to forgive all. In spiritual practice one is taught to forgive others; in psychotherapy one learns to forgive oneself. Both are necessary for complete forgiveness and well-being.

7. Love. Psychotherapy and spiritual practice can both lead to opening the heart and developing the capacity to give and receive love. Spirituality awakens the awareness of love's presence in our lives; psychotherapy cultivates love in relationship.

8. Awareness. Depth psychotherapy and spiritual practice both cultivate awareness and non-judgmental attention. A therapist who helps clients develop self-awareness can benefit from a meditation practice that enhances sensitivity to nuances of experience.

9. Liberation. Both psychotherapy and spiritual practice can contribute to liberation from limiting self-concepts. Freedom from fear and delusion, from the past, and from early conditioning are common goals.

> *Becoming human means discovering our fullness and learning to live from it. This involves bringing forth more of who we really are and becoming more available to whatever life presents.*
>
> JOHN WELWOOD

RESOURCES

Books

Benner, D. G. *Psychotherapy and the Spiritual Quest.* Grand Rapids, MI: Baker Book House, 1988.

Grof, S., ed. *Ancient Wisdom and Modern Science.* New York: SUNY Press, 1984.

Nelson, J. E. *Healing the Split: Madness or Transcendence?* Los Angeles: J. P. Tarcher, 1990.

Wilber, K. *The Spectrum of Consciousness.* Wheaton, IL: Theosophical Publishing House, 1977.

————, J. Engler, and D. P. Brown, eds. *Transformations of Consciousness: Conventional and Contemplative Perspectives on Development.* Boston, MA: Shambhala, 1986.

Periodicals

The Common Boundary, published bimonthly, is aimed at healing and helping professionals interested in exploring the interface between psychotherapy and spirituality. The subscription address is: 8528 Bradford Road, Silver Spring, MD 20901.

KUNDALINI AWAKENING: BREAKDOWN OR BREAKTHROUGH?
BY STUART SOVATSKY, PH.D.

What the woman was describing so excitedly over the phone was a kundalini awakening. Not all awakenings of the body's psychospiritual energy are experienced as similarly benign. In some cases, they can involve all kinds of psychological and physical problems. In discussing some of the pitfalls on the spiritual path, however, I should begin with a note of encouragement, lest the kundalini's reputation as dangerous gain too much prominence. As with anything "unusual," the positive or negative quality of this experience may hinge on one's interpretation. The clinic's co-founder, psychiatrist Lee Sannella, M.D., addressed this ambiguity in the title of his book, *The Kundalini Experience: Transcendence or Psychosis?* For the individual, the question is an immediate one: Are these heated tingles, images of death and rebirth, uncanny synchronicities, mood swings, and unusual perceptual phenomena breakthroughs or breakdowns in consciousness? Answering this question is not merely a matter of nomenclature; it is the first thing one "does" to the experience, and perhaps the most crucial.

If I accept my sensations as a breakthrough, they will be experienced initially as pleasurable. But if the experience then intensifies to the point of discomfort, I may begin to resist the sensations, which in turn generates fear. As Sannella notes, "A schizophrenia-like condition can result when the person undergoing the kundalini experience receives negative feedback either from social pressure or from the resistance of his or her earlier conditioning." Interpreting the difficulty as a "punishment," I may plummet into guilt, until I can relax and gradually sense some overriding, protective ambience or grace. Thus, the process continues, varying from moment to moment as my reactions also vary. I may feel like Jonah before the whale, St. Francis in the woods, or the

161

When Kundalini is awakened and this more potent energy goes to the brain, our consciousness at once undergoes a transformation.

GOPI KRISHNA

most insignificant speck in the cosmos. Yet, when experience and experiencer merge in a transcendental trust, what then matters? These are the moments of enlightenment scattered like wildflowers throughout the wondrous and tumultuous journey.

For the past 20 years, the work of the Kundalini Clinic has been to support people through such difficult and transformative experiences. When I am on the phone with an anxious caller or in the clinic with a confused client, the clinician's diagnostic question—is this person psychotic or in the process of an awakening?—is displaced by the immediate need to help the client feel safe, understood, and accepted. Thus, the earlier goal of the clinic—to distinguish between psychosis and kundalini awakening—has been reshaped into providing drug-free, hospital-free treatment for people who might otherwise receive more intrusive forms of therapy. This broadened goal is a natural outgrowth of the original work of the clinic, which now treats individuals undergoing a wide range of personal and relational crises.

Psychosis, which is defined as a "gross impairment of reality testing," usually occurs without kundalini awakening. The symptoms of psychosis that distinguish it from such awakening include a greater degree of dissociation, inward preoccupation with paranoid feelings, and usually less ability to communicate directly with others. The kundalini experience may generate what psychiatry would call hallucinations, but these psychic phenomena tend to be less threatening than those experienced in psychosis and indeed may appear beneficent. Although psychotic experiences often involve unusual body sensations, they rarely include the ineffable bliss or the heated tingles felt in the chakra sites stimulated by pranic or kundalini energy.

At the Kundalini Clinic, however, both experiences are seen as an opportunity for growth. All unusual, bizarre, or "crazy" symptoms are treated as meaningful expressions of some internal, perhaps convoluted drive toward wholeness. When this meaning is discovered and therapeutically integrated into the client's world, greater wholeness or ego strength is achieved. When ordinary reality appears transitory and illusory, as it does in both kundalini and psychotic experiences, what are we to say and do? Call it psychosis and prescribe appropriate medications? Perhaps we can only say that the ego, the mentality that labels and contains ordinary reality, must inevitably surrender to primal mysteries such as kundalini, or to the internal and external factors that provide the psychotic break.

The clinic often attracts people who do not want to join an

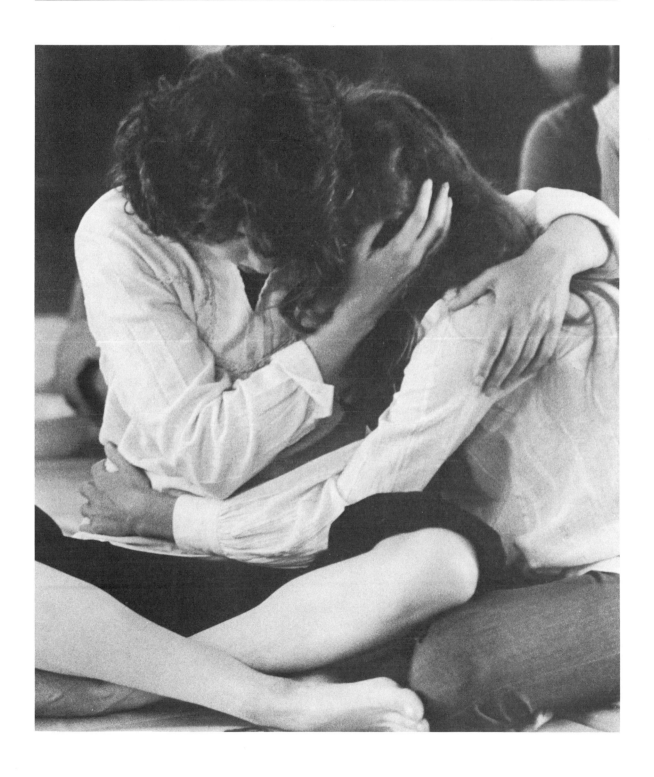

organized spiritual group and may have been practicing spiritual disciplines on their own for some time. Coming to the clinic may be a first step toward adopting a more conventional, socially integrated lifestyle, or toward dealing with psychological issues that recur despite meditative progress. Clients may be looking for confirmation or recognition of their highly unusual, idiosyncratic experiences.

One woman's energetic awakening was covered over by congenital cerebral palsy. After identifying the awakening, she practiced certain breathing techniques and was able to decrease her spasticity and develop greater self-acceptance. Another client's awakening was complicated by the trauma of being an unwanted child, which blocked her emotional expression. In therapy she tearfully relived those early experiences, thereby dissolving the blocks. Others say jogging or a traumatic illness triggered the "strange experiences" that prompted them to call the Kundalini Clinic.

In keeping with co-founder Dr. Harold Streitfeld's discovery that body-based psychotherapy helps resolve the repetitive kriyas (involuntary body movements) generated by kundalini activity, the clinic offers Reichian therapy and yogic techniques along with the more verbal psychotherapies. The goal is to keep using the intensified state of mind to examine one's life and relationships and to continue to explore paranormal and spiritual dimensions. All clients at the clinic who have experienced kundalini awakening have voiced a strong desire to channel their heightened energies into socially useful activities, such as revived commitment to parenthood, professional training in psychological or physical therapies, original nutritional research, or work in the fine arts.

The process of positively interpreting the symptoms constituting the "kundalini syndrome" can be viewed as a kind of "informed faith healing." For example, if one is puzzled by a certain burning, tingling sensation in the spine, accurate information about purificatory "pranic movements" can be very reassuring. Of course, to believe that such pranic movements are being guided by a beneficent, superconscious intelligence requires faith. And finding "grounds" for such faith may become the crux of the relationship between the individual and his or her experience.

Ultimately, kundalini activity challenges us to stretch and test our capacity to integrate new and perhaps difficult experiences while "keeping the faith." As the purification becomes more complete, we discover that all of existence is an outpouring of divine manifestation. When this insight persists without ego inflation, we must agree that an enlightenment has occurred.

To identify with the ego is to confuse the organism with its history.

ALAN W. WATTS

Resources

Books

Bragdon, E. *The Call of Spiritual Emergency.* San Francisco: HarperSan-Francisco, 1989.

Grof, C., and S. Grof. *The Stormy Search for the Self: A Guide to Personal Growth through Transformational Crisis.* Los Angeles: J. P. Tarcher, 1990.

Grof, S., and C. Grof, eds. *Spiritual Emergency: When Personal Transformation Becomes a Crisis.* Los Angeles: J. P. Tarcher, 1989.

Sannella, L. *The Kundalini Experience: Transcendence or Psychosis?* Lower Lake, CA: Integral Publishing, 2nd ed., 1987.

Periodicals

Friends in New Directions (F.I.N.D.) Newsletter, c/o E. Holland, R.R. 5 Flesherton, Ontario, Canada NOC 1EO.

Organizations

The Kundalini Clinic, directed by Stuart Sovatsky, Ph.D., 3040 Richmond Boulevard, Oakland, CA 94611. Tel. (510) 465-2986.

The Kundalini Research Foundation, P.O. Box 2248, Darian, CT 06820. Tel. (203) 348-5351.

Spiritual Emergence Network (SEN) provides information for people undergoing transformational crises and acts as a referral service. It is located at 5905 Soquel #650, Soquel, CA 95073. Tel. (510) 464-8261.

What Makes Spiritual Teachers Go Astray?
by Diana Leafe Christian

"Guru hit by sex-slave suit," clamors the headline in the *San Francisco Examiner.* We have all probably heard or read of at least one such accusation or exposé of amassed wealth, violence, alcoholism, or sexual misconduct—activities that may be commonplace among politicos and foreign dictators but seem incomprehensible in those individuals who are here to help us transcend all that.

Assuming that at least some of these exposés are true, *why* would a supposedly enlightened master begin behaving so badly? Was he or she an imposter from the outset? Are many Western seekers just fools?

Another Look at "Enlightenment"

To explore this issue, I suggest we take a fresh look at many commonly held assumptions about spiritual teachers and attempt, if we can, to understand the "occupational hazards" to which a guru is subject.

Are "divine lila" or "crazy wisdom" valid explanations for erratic behavior?

These terms refer to the enlightened teacher's behaving in "crazy," inexplicable ways, which are said to actually teach the student and further his or her spiritual progress or serve some function in a yet-to-be-revealed "divine plan." Assuming for the moment that the teacher *does* know what is best for the student (or the plan), the question becomes:

Is our teacher really enlightened, and what makes us think so?

We get this belief primarily from Asian devotees and meditators, and they get it from their culture and scriptures. Texts tell us to rely completely on our "spiritual friend," to unquestioningly obey the roshi, to put all our faith in the lama's enlightenment, to view the yogi as identical to the deity, and even to worship the guru with ardent devotion, for the quality of our *bhakti* will determine the outcome of our spiritual progress. Even in those traditions where the teacher is not revered as a god-like figure, he or she is at least viewed as an accomplished meditator and guide on the path, to be honored and *trusted*.

Do we know what "enlightened" means anyway?

If we were to ask ten committed Western practitioners of an Eastern spiritual discipline what "enlightenment" is, we would probably receive ten very different answers. The reason for this multiplicity of beliefs, I feel, is that each major tradition defines the state somewhat differently, as does each school or sect within that tradition and, often, each lineage within each school or sect as well. Some sources describe an either-or situation: you *are* enlightened or you are *not* enlightened; others relate a continuum of ever-higher stages or levels of consciousness, whose number and description vary from source to source. At the pinnacle of each continuum, however, is an "enlightenment" that is deemed permanent, irreversible.

Man has always stood in need of spiritual help.

C. G. JUNG

166

Besides tradition, what else convinces us that our teacher is "enlightened"? And are we qualified to judge?

For one thing, our personal experiences convince us. Many students have had blissfully transcendent or supernatural experiences in the presence of their teacher. These experiences are so unlike anything else that they may have encountered that they can only conclude their teacher is a master of the highest order. But does it really mean that?

Do siddhis and charisma a master make?

I once knew a charming, radiant, charismatic teacher who successfully taught most of his small following to connect clairaudiently with the "higher Self" so they could better receive inner advice and become calm and centered at will. The teacher had remarkable powers. He was clairaudient, and sometimes clairvoyant. He claimed to call on angelic beings for wisdom and healings, and several followers were indeed healed. He claimed to experience ecstatic communion with these beings for days on end and would emerge from his retreats more radiant than usual, almost visibly surrounded by light. On several occasions I and several others observed him insert large needles through the skin of his cheeks and arms without pain or bleeding, and chew up and swallow razor blades with no apparent harm.

This teacher believed that stressful confrontations were useful in helping his students to evoke the higher Self. He therefore collected "collateral"—the student's most prized possession—to be forfeited if the student did not obey him implicitly. He then took groups of students on hikes and threatened to hurl one or two of them off a cliff if they didn't summon their higher Selves and become immediately calm. As a further confrontation, he would ask students to masturbate in front of the group. And as an ultimate confront, he would ask students (both male and female) to engage in one or another sexual activity with him. When they finally agreed (perhaps remembering the collateral), the teacher would either withdraw the request or go through with it, sometimes in the presence of other group members. After a trip to his own guru in India, the teacher set up his modest home as an ashram for students, with himself, not the Indian, as the figurehead.

What are we to make of this? I believe that a teacher can develop awesome power (shakti) and impressive paranormal abilities (siddhis) and still not be enlightened. Or infallible. Many people assume that their experiences prove their teacher to be a realized master, or at least very advanced spiritually. But consider the possibility that this belief is a specious one, and that the leap of faith from the experience to the conclusion is unwarranted. An adept can develop marvelous—even transferrable—spiritual abilities, but still not be beyond errors of judgment or action. And as the story of the razor blade yogi illustrates, having charisma and siddhis does not mean one is advanced spiritually or has even resolved all power or sexual issues—it is proof of nothing more than having developed charisma and siddhis.

Indian psychoanalyst Dr. Sudhir Kakar emphasizes this point in his book *Shamans, Mystics, and Doctors*, paraphrasing the Austrian-born mystic and professor of anthropology Agehananda Bharati:

> Mysticism is a skill that can be learned. Its practice leads to an achievement (the mystical experience) which neither confers supernatural powers or superhuman status on the practitioner nor imbues him with any moral excellence beyond what he can acquire through accompanying efforts of a nonmystical kind: moral, artistic, intellectual. The widespread Indian belief to the contrary, there is little evidence that the mystic is somehow a "better" human being because of his mystical efforts and experience. Indeed, some of the best-known mystics have been and continue to be pompous and self-righteous, woman-haters and politically fascist.[4]

An increasingly prevalent belief is the idea that if we experience something personally, it must be so. Many of us who have been influenced by the human potential movement revere "experience" as sacrosanct, perhaps forgetting the possibility that perceptions can be distorted by an unconscious agenda or lack of sufficient information.

But in the case of spiritual teachers, who can really blame us? We have nothing in our cultural context in which to place them. Our cultural naiveté might be compared to the reactions of a house guest from Delhi who is watching American television for the first time. Suddenly young Gopal leaps from the couch and runs to us, breathless and excited.

"Oh, we must come on down to Wide Track Town! Mr. Harry has actually *slashed* the prices on his used Pontiacs, and they will remain slashed for the next three hours only!"

Of course we would burst out laughing. We are all so used to Harry's used-car commercials we don't even hear them anymore, but

A preceptor who confounds spirituality with occultism indeed misses the incomparable sweetness of the former and is like a goat which devours the sugar-cane leaves and leaves the sugar-cane behind.

SWAMI GNANANANDA

Gopal (who has always yearned for an American car) is beside himself with fervor.

Similarly, an educated and well-traveled Hindu does not salivate at the news of a new *baba* in town. The Indian places the information in its cultural context and asks, "Who is the fellow, and who are his devotees? What is his lineage? Who was his teacher? What does he teach? Who has he helped? Can he cure Uncle Rajendra's indigestion?"

It also might be wise, if not humbling, to consider that most of us are probably not already "enlightened" ourselves and presumably cannot ascertain the level, or stability, of another being's spiritual attainment. Just as the precision of a neurosurgeon's work can be evaluated only by another neurosurgeon, it takes a master to know a master. Elisabeth Haich, for example, a renowned European Yoga teacher and author of *Initiation*, believes a master can only be recognized and understood by someone on a spiritual level very near his or her own.[5]

So What Makes Gurus Run Amok?

What happens to make a spiritually accomplished and perhaps enlightened individual behave so erratically? Can enlightenment, once gained, be lost?

1. Least likely, I think, is that the teacher is a calculating phony with a taste for power, fame, and baksheesh.

2. The teacher is deluded but very sincere, fooled by the evidence of rapturous states, paranormal abilities, and impressive powers. With no watchful master to set things straight, the guru goes off to teach, motivated partly out of a heartfelt desire to serve and partly out of unquenched longings for wealth and prestige.

3. The teacher has reached a high level of spiritual development but has overlooked subconscious emotional conflicts, which, though unobservable to the ordinary person, continue to exert an influence in subtle ways.

4. The teacher has reached a level of actual enlightenment (however defined), but is still "stained" by perceptible remnants of individual ego.

In these last two scenarios, if the teacher stays home with his or her master and meditates, the unconscious issues will hopefully be brought

Everybody has his own path, his mission, and even if you take your Master as a model, you must always develop in the way that suits your own nature. You have to sing the part which has been given to you, aware of the notes, the beat, and the rhythm; you have to sing it with your voice, which is certainly not that of your Master, but that is not important. The one really important thing is to sing your part perfectly.

OMRAAM MIKHAEL AIVANHOV

to light and transmuted, and any last remnants of illusion will eventually be released.

But what if the teacher goes off to the West? Any unresolved issues of power or sexuality or subtle vestiges of ego may become snagged on the abrasive edges of American life, tragically unravelling lifetimes of diligent effort. (Many of these same temptations could seduce an American-born teacher as well.)

Strangers in a strange land. Imagine for a moment that you are such a guru. Imbued with the Divine Presence or the Clear and Radiant Void, blissfully content, filled with compassion for others, you step off the plane into the land of supermarkets and credit cards.

Everywhere you turn you are met with unprecedented technical virtuosity and material abundance. You are assailed by the pervasive "be sexual" campaign waged by Madison Avenue, Hollywood, and popular culture. You are not respected by the majority of citizens because you are perceived as an Asian foreigner in funny robes, and, worse yet, you pose a potential threat to the hold the traditional religions hope to keep over the nation's youth. Nor are your spiritual attainments respected, or even recognized, for the most part.

Of course, you soon have followers who love and respect you, but because of your cultural isolation they are virtually the only people with whom you interact. These followers can raise money with surprising alacrity. It doesn't take long before your organization has a center, then a network of centers, regularly scheduled teachings, a printing press. You write books; you are interviewed in the alternative press. You have more and more students, and access to undreamed-of sums of money.

Unlike women in your own country, your female students may not have been raised to be modest or demure or to keep a respectful distance from religious figures. If you are a man, they may have a frank sexual interest in you; they may even fall in love with you. Their feelings are transparent, palpable.

You are certain, however, that neither the materially rich culture nor your libido-rich students can detract from your awareness of effulgent Reality or your unswerving devotion to service. The suffering Occidentals are numberless; you vow to enlighten them all.

But you cannot see your blind spots. And your teacher is not here to guide you.

Accepting projection. According to some sources, teachers can be subtly or profoundly influenced (depending on their degree of spiritual

If any human guru is giving you teachings that bring you closer in your heart to the Divine, listen and be grateful and follow them. But be clear about the limitations of all human gurus.

MOTHER MEERA

attainment) by the emotional projections of their followers. Dr. Kakar, who like many of his countrymen is as skeptical of gurus as Americans are of used-car salesmen, believes devotees idealize and "uncritically eulogize" their gurus beyond any merit the teachers naturally possess. The devotees do this, he says, so they may identify with a special, superior being, because—in addition to whatever spiritual advantage they may gain—it feels so comforting to have a superhuman as a parent-substitute.

Because the flattering projections are "narcissistically gratifying," he says, the teacher accepts them as reality and becomes ego-inflated, however unconsciously. "To be consistently thought greater, more wonderful, and more intelligent than we are," he says, "is a burden only in the sense that one may feel impelled to be greater, more wonderful and intelligent. . . . Most often . . . the guru simply accepts these projections as belonging to his self and enters into unconscious collusion with the followers—'I am uncannily sensitive, infinitely wise, miraculously powerful; you are not.'"[6]

This opinion seems a bit harsh and is certainly limited by the concepts of psychoanalysis, but it does provide one explanation for what may contribute to the downfall of those teachers who left their native lands carrying subtle ego needs as excess baggage.

Although the phenomenon is not scientifically observable, a very similar description exists in the literature of Western metaphysicians, who claim that when followers have strong feelings about a teacher, an emotionally charged "thought form" can be created out of their collective non-physical, "astral" substance. Such a thought form is said to attain cohesive, quasi-conscious status and literally hovers around the teacher and group. British metaphysician Dion Fortune explains the phenomena in more psychological terms: "When a number of people have their attention focused on the same object . . . and feel toward this object the same emotion, . . . the free-floating portions of [the group's] subconsciousness tend to flow together and amalgamate in a single cloud."[7] This "cloud" profoundly affects the emotions of the group and teacher, she says.

It seems unlikely that an emotional "group mind," if it really existed, could have much impact on a highly realized adept, but again, for a teacher with unfinished ego business, such a creation might prove one more contributor to his or her undoing.

Blowing a fuse. Some metaphysicians speculate that another source of potential trouble for a teacher has to do, paradoxically, with the

To find a living guru is a rare opportunity and a great responsibility.

SRI NISARGADATTA
MAHARAJ

It is the disciple that makes the guru great.

SRI NISARGADATTA
MAHARAJ

unusually high levels of spiritual energy the teacher is said to channel through his or her body. (Again, this theory is based not on any measurable laboratory test, but on what a wide spectrum of Western clairvoyants claim to "see" when they observe allegedly nonphysical energy dynamics taking place within and between individuals.)

Many such observers, including Fortune and Elisabeth Haich, claim living beings are composed of various frequencies of energy that are circulated through their physical and non-physical bodies. Accomplished masters, they say, have consciously transmuted their grosser consciousness—and therefore their energies—into ever-higher frequencies and operate on an energy level far more refined and highly charged than that of the average person. The problem arises, Haich and Fortune point out, when a teacher is not absolutely stable in the transformation of these energies, as when, to use a common metaphor, a wire is not strong enough to contain an ever-increasing voltage.

Yang and yin *are deadly enemies who need one another.*

C. G. JUNG

These energy frequencies are dual in nature, the theory goes, and are described in the West as "negatively" or "positively" charged, and in the East as yin and yang or Shakti and Shiva energies. Each individual, it is said, contains both polarities; males are polarized predominantly with "positive," yang energy, and females with "negative," yin energy.

The dynamic interplay between these polarities is supposedly responsible for the active functioning of both sexual and spiritual energies. In fact, sexual and spiritual energies are, according to many Western metaphysical schools and some Eastern spiritual teachings, actually different harmonics of the same basic divine force. For instance, solitary meditators, often monks and nuns, have reported strong sexual arousal, with no apparent cause, while in meditative states; and couples with no particular interest in spiritual pursuits have reported overpoweringly transcendent, spiritual experiences while making love.[8]

If a yogi, through long years of meditative practice and guidance, creates powerful enough channels (in Sanskrit *nadis*) to safely contain these energies, all is well. If this growth process is interrupted, however, and the channels are not fully developed, the energies may leap out and "ground" themselves in someone with an opposite polarity. This instability of the energies coursing through the channels—and their urge to burst their bounds—will be experienced as overwhelming *sexual* desire.

Fortune writes of this process in the case of a male teacher:

The greater cosmic forces . . . will be very apt to make a path of returning for themselves through any conductile vehicle that approaches sufficiently close, leaping the gap like an electric spark; and if the individual who receives the force be of insufficient calibre to carry the voltage, her emotional nature will . . . fuse, and there will be an open circuit of cosmic forces which will also fuse the positive or male vehicle, burn all in their immediate neighbourhood, and break the contact with Divine forces.[9]

In other words, the master will blow a fuse. Fortune emphatically believes that such an individual has suffered an accident of *energy* rather than a lapse of morality:

It was a spiritual force that broke the bounds, and not a force of the underworld. The tremendous cosmic energy which that man had caused to flow through the channel of his individualized self proved of greater voltage . . . than he could carry, and so his spiritual nature fused under the strain and "short circuited." . . . He was as little culpable as is the man whose mill-dam gives way and swamps a village.[10]

Of course, psychoanalytic speculation and clairvoyant observations don't prove anything, but these ideas may shed some light on the sad phenomenon of guru demise. Perhaps we who read shocking headlines or exposé magazine articles of suddenly renegade masters can better understand the special pressures with which a guru is beset and can muster a bit of that same compassion that motivates so many teachers to take on students in the first place.

The Flow of Empowerment

Many who have read this far may well be thinking, "This may be true for some gurus, but it has nothing to do with *my* teacher!" And I can't blame you; I feel the same way about my own teacher, who certainly seems to evidence an abundance of sweetness, gentle gaiety, and inner stillness. Since most of us (I presume) are faced with the interesting paradox of not being enlightened enough ourselves to recognize a fully enlightened master when we see one, the best rule of thumb, I think, is to apply a healthy dose of what Mahayana Buddhists call "discriminating awareness" (Sanskrit *prajna*; Tibetan *shes-rab*).

We also might do well to keep an eye on which way the empowerment flows. If empowerment, expressed as blessings, nurturance, and wisdom, flows primarily from the teacher to ourselves, and we feel increasingly nourished, whole, and compassionate as a result, then

The function of the teacher is indeed an affair of the transference of something, and not one of mere stimulation of the existing intellectual or other faculties in the taught.

SWAMI VIVEKANANDA

probably all is well. But if the empowerment flows primarily from our-selves to the teacher, in whatever form, and we begin to feel weakened, defensive, or confused, we may have cause for concern.

RESOURCES

Books

When a teaching is turned into a cult and congealed into a sect, it is time to get up and go away.

PAUL BRUNTON

Anthony, D., B. Ecker, and K. Wilber, eds. *Spiritual Choices: The Problem of Recognizing Authentic Paths to Inner Transformation.* New York: Paragon House, 1987. An important treatment of cults and genuine spirituality.

Feuerstein, G. *Holy Madness: The Shock Tactics and Radical Teachings of Crazy-Wise Adepts, Holy Fools, and Rascal Gurus.* New York: Paragon House, 1991. An in-depth study of teachers and spiritual discipleship in many traditions, including contemporary schools and cults.

Nisker, S. *Crazy Wisdom.* Berkeley, CA: Ten Speed Press, 1990. An anthology-type treatment of the extraordinary teachings and teaching styles of spiritual adepts around the world, meant to inform and en-tertain.

Vaughan, F. *The Inward Arc: Healing and Wholeness in Psychotherapy and Spirituality.* Boston: Shambhala, 1986. A highly readable book contain-ing sound insights on the interface between psychological well-being and spirituality.

EARLY-WARNING SIGNS
FOR THE DETECTION OF SPIRITUAL BLIGHT
BY DANIEL GOLEMAN, PH.D.

Spiritual groups—like families, corporations, therapy groups, and marriages—are susceptible to the full range of human foibles. Vanity, power-seeking, and looking out for Number One are as likely to show up in a spiritual organization as any other. The very nature of such groups often makes it difficult to notice or acknowledge that something is awry. Group collusions, such as "It's all part of the Teaching," are in-voked to alibi for meanness of spirit and pettiness.

Wandering the spiritual path by no means protects us from the nor-mal dose of folly that accompanies any other human endeavor. Spiritual work is perhaps all the more ripe for foibles because of the excellent cover-up that self-deception lends for the use of the spirit in the service of the ego, libido, and pocketbook.

As a spiritual freelancer for many years who has been at the center or periphery of a variety of such groups, I have had ample opportunity to note or fall prey to some of the typical pitfalls listed below. Of course, in one or another context each of these signals may be a false negative—a benign symptom with no underlying pathology. More often than not, they mean that an open-minded, skeptical enquiry is called for.

Be wary when you notice the first signs of:

Taboo topics. Questions that can't be asked, doubts that can't be shared, misgivings that can't be voiced. For example, "Where does all the money go?" or "Does yogi sleep with his secretary?"

Secrets. The suppression of information, usually tightly guarded by an inner circle. For example, the answers, "Swiss bank accounts," or "Yes, he does—and that's why she had an abortion."

Spiritual clones. In its minor form, stereotypic behavior, such as people who walk, talk, smoke, eat, and dress just like their leader; in its more sinister form, psychological stereotyping, such as an entire group of people who manifest only a narrow range of feeling in any and all situations; always happy, or pious, or reduce everything to a single explanation, or sardonic, etc.

Groupthink. A party line that overrides how people actually feel. Typically the cognitive glue that binds the group. For example, "You're fallen, and Christ is the answer"; or "You're impure, and Shiva is the answer."

The elect. A shared delusion of grandeur that there is no Way but this one. The corollary: you're lost if you leave the group.

No graduates. Members are never weaned from the group. Often accompanies the corollary above.

Assembly lines. Everyone is treated identically, no matter what their differences; e.g., mantras assigned by dictates of a demographical checklist.

Loyalty tests. Members are asked to prove loyalty to the group by doing something that violates their personal ethics; for example, set up an organization that has a hidden agenda of recruiting others into the group but publicly represents itself as a public service outfit.

Duplicity. The group's public face misrepresents its true nature, as in the example just given.

Unifocal understanding. A single world view is used to explain anything and everything; alternate explanations are verboten. For example, if you have diarrhea it's "Guru's Grace." If it stops, it's also Guru's Grace. And if you get constipated, it's still Guru's Grace.

The house of the Divine is not closed to any who knock sincerely at its gates, whatever their past stumbles and errors.

SRI AUROBINDO

A teacher should have maximal authority, and minimal power.

THOMAS SZASZ

Humorlessness. No irreverence allowed. Laughing at sacred cows is good for your health. Take, for example, Gurdjieff's one-liner: "If you want to lose your faith, make friends with a priest."

GUIDEPOSTS ON THE PATH
BY STEPHAN BODIAN

Through doubt we arrive at the truth.

CICERO

The spiritual path makes paradoxical demands on us. It bids us set aside our limited, habitual ways of perceiving things in order to cultivate our innate potential to perceive reality directly. In the meantime, we are caught between certainties—the old ones are in ruins, the new ones loom on the distant horizon like a tantalizing mirage. And hanging out in the valley of uncertainty, where things are no longer as they once appeared, we are exceptionally vulnerable to the lies, half-truths, and rationalizations of powerful authority figures (and their followers) who claim to possess higher wisdom but who may in fact be more "endarkened" than we are.

How do we proceed? Do we spurn spiritual practice entirely? Or do we keep one foot out the door in case we need to beat a hasty retreat? What about issues of trust and surrender, which figure so prominently on the spiritual path but also leave us open to possible exploitation? Here I would like to offer some guidelines to help fellow seekers negotiate the trackless terrain that has rather euphemistically been called the spiritual "path."

1. **Trust your common sense and your intuition.** They are the only reliable equipment you have for navigating in this flawed phenomenal universe of ours. The thinking mind can be put to sleep by lofty sermonizing, but there is a deeper place, in the gut, where you know exactly what's going on.

2. **Feel free to question and to doubt.** When asked about unscrupulous teachers, His Holiness the Dalai Lama replies that Westerners are too quick to surrender. In the Tibetan tradition, he says, students spend years with a teacher observing his behavior, questioning others about him, noting whether he lives the principles he teaches, before deciding to take him on as a guru. Indeed, in the early years of practice, students are encouraged to doubt both teachers and teachings.

3. **Keep your wits about you.** This guideline is a corollary of the last. The intellect may be easily bamboozled, but it sure comes in handy

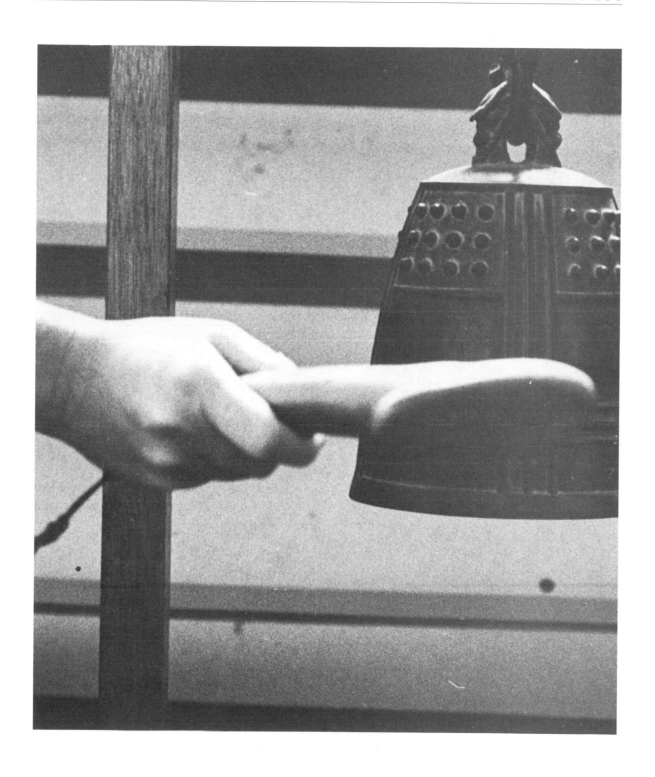

when trying to sort out conflicting messages or make sense of a confusing relationship or group involvement. Beware of hidden persuasions and other attempts to take advantage of others by bypassing the rational mind in the name of some higher value, like love or devotion. The great spiritual traditions have a place for the intellect, rather than denouncing or suppressing it.

Revering the master is not enough. Having faith in the master is an elementary beginning. Fervent admiration may provoke interest, but it will not effect transformation. The master does not need praise. He desires his disciples' actualization of their inherent capacities.

JUSTIN O'BRIEN

4. Maintain firm boundaries. Those of us who grew up in unhealthy families (90 percent of the population, some experts say) didn't realize we had a right to say no. Because we were taught that our parents were always right, we assumed they must have good reason when they shamed us or beat us or sexually abused us. As adults, we lack what psychologists call healthy boundaries: a clear sense of our inalienable rights as human beings to privacy, to our own feelings and ideas, to our own bodies. Don't relinquish your right to say no.

5. Take your time. Here again, the Dalai Lama gives apt advice. Don't rush into a spiritual involvement, any more than you'd rush into a marriage. Listen to the resistant, skeptical parts of yourself—they may hold insights the rest of you ignores.

6. Enlightenment is no substitute for doing your karmic homework. I have met too many so-called enlightened masters with shadows longer than their entourage to believe that a profound experience of truth is any more than just that. After the dust has settled and the stars have fallen from the eyes, you are left with the lifelong task of transforming old, stubborn patterns of perceiving and behaving into openness, spontaneity, beginner's mind. "Situations are the best teachers," Chogyam Trungpa was fond of saying. So are spouses, children, parents, bosses, friends.

7. Learn more about family and group dysfunction. The videos and books of psychologist John Bradshaw should be required viewing and reading for all spiritual practitioners. Informal polls of ashrams and zendos reveal that a disproportionate number of inhabitants come from alcoholic or otherwise severely dysfunctional families.

8. Sex with a spiritual teacher is never in the student's best interest. The authors of the book *Spiritual Choices* articulate and then proceed to demolish three arguments often advanced to explain why a spiritual teacher might justifiably engage in sexual relations with disciples. Their conclusion is that a "master who sexually exploits a trusting disciple is comparable to a parent who molests a child."

9. Siddhis do not a guru make. Special powers (siddhis) can be most impressive, as can a teacher's charisma or air of authority, but they have little if anything to do with the qualities of wisdom and compassion, which are the primary marks of an enlightened person. Don't be impressed by psychic powers or other extraordinary abilities—they are just as likely to be used to benefit a big ego as to serve others.

10. The true guru is inside you. The guru out there is just a projection of all the wonderful virtues we possess as our birthright and only need to actualize. And the ultimate authority, the master, the source, abides nowhere but in our own hearts.

The new spiritual man will not be man converted to Proclus or Buddha, but man within whom they, and also Moses and Christ and Faust, can coexist more comfortably than before—though not necessarily with equal value.

ROBERT S. ELLWOOD

Notes

[1] A. Huxley, *The Perennial Philosophy* (New York: Harper, 1944), p. vii.

[2] A. Maslow, *Toward a Psychology of Being* (New York: Van Nostrand, 1968), pp. iii–iv.

[3] K. Wilber, *No Boundary: Eastern and Western Approaches to Personal Growth* (Boston, MA: New Science Library, 1980), p. 4.

[4] S. Kakar, *Shamans, Mystics, and Doctors* (Boston, MA: Beacon Press, 1982), p. 122.

[5] E. Haich, *Sexual Energy and Yoga* (New York: ASI Publishers, 1972), p. 90.

[6] S. Kakar, *op. cit.*, pp. 149–150.

[7] D. Fortune, *Esoteric Philosophy of Love and Marriage* (New York: Weiser, 1967), p. 48.

[8] D. U. Neff, "The Divine Embrace," *Yoga Journal*, March–April 1982; "Tantra: A Tradition Unveiled," *Yoga Journal*, January–February and March–April, 1983.

[9] D. Fortune, *op. cit.*, pp. 69–70.

[10] Ibid., pp. 37, 38.

PART THREE

CULTIVATING LOVE:
BHAKTI YOGA

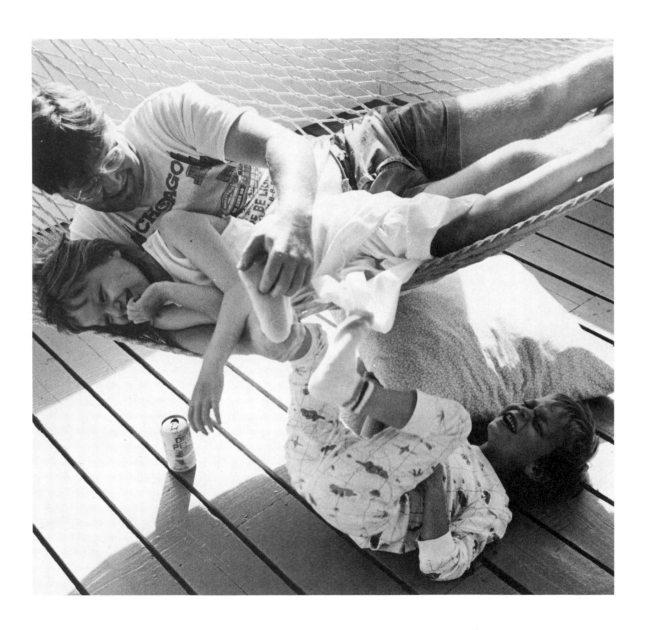

NINE

The Journey of the Heart

THE RADIANT FORCE OF LOVE

The contributions in this chapter all deal with various applications of bhakti yoga, the way of the heart, or the spiritual discipline of love. As we have seen in Chapter 6, love is a great healing force. Here we will examine how love can be consciously cultivated to harmonize and uplift our personal relationships so that they can serve the spiritual process of self-discovery and self-transcendence.

An important expression of love is sexuality—an area of conflict and frustration for many people, though it need not be. Thus one of the essays in this chapter proposes that sexuality and spirituality are not contradictory forms of self-expression, but that the sexual drive can be employed to heighten our level of psychosomatic energy and to intensify our spiritual awareness. This approach is based on the ancient ideal of sacred sexuality.

Another essay looks at voluntary celibacy as a powerful antidote to the modern sexual malaise. Celibacy, it is argued, can greatly enhance the life force within us.

Whether you wish to experiment with a celibate lifestyle or remain sexually active, the practice of bhakti yoga is as relevant today as it was thousands of years ago. By inviting the sacred into our hearts and into our most intimate relationships, we are able to actively transform our lives and align them more and more with the great universal ideals of yoga.

Love of self, desire, erotic passion, the need for friendship, tenderness between parents and children— this is the raw material. These feelings are redirected toward an ideal or a divinity . . . and their energy acts as a propelling force for the ascent toward the transpersonal stratosphere.

PIERO FERRUCCI

"Love, and do what you will." These words of St. Augustine character-
ize the approach of bhakti yoga, which draws on our innate ability to
be all-embracing. When we truly love, we are in harmony not only with
our beloved but with all living things. Love is blind, insofar as it makes
no distinctions but extends to everyone and everything.

A common Sanskrit word for "love" is *bhakti*, which stems from the
verbal root *bhaj*, meaning "to participate." Love is the most profound
participation of which we are capable. We are in touch with the very
essence of all others. As Westerners, we may have difficulty in grasping
this notion, for we have become accustomed to using the word "love"
interchangeably with "liking," and in just about any situation.

When we love someone, we may well like her beauty and charm or
his good looks and wit. However, what we love, if we truly love, cannot
be catalogued in this fashion, because it concerns a person's indefinable
spiritual essence. Since that essence is the same in all of us, genuine
love is unqualified. So, love also includes the desire to merge completely, which is indeed the condition of our spiritual essence, the transcendental Self (*atman*). At the highest level of existence, we are all
united. Hindu scriptures refer to this supreme condition as the joyous
union between Shiva (the masculine cosmic principle) and Shakti (the
feminine cosmic principle).

Our natural state, prior to the appearance of the individuated
body-mind, is one of love and bliss. Our feelings of personal love, compassion, empathy, reverence, and devotion are manifestations of that
deeper love-bliss. Bhakti yoga makes use of these positive human emotions, to help us awaken to our true identity and recover the original
love-bliss. It seeks to refine them until our ability to love extends into
infinity.

*These two teachings—the
supremacy of the heart and the
uniqueness of each human being
are very important to me. They
give me the fullest understanding
of my membership in the human
family.*

ROBERT MULLER

RESOURCES

Books

Andrews, F. *The Art and Practice of Loving*. New York: J. P. Tarcher/
Perigee, 1992.

Buscaglia, L. *Love*. New York: Fawcett Crest, 1972.

Cooey, P. M., et al., eds. *Embodied Love: Sensuality and Relationship as Femi-
nist Values*. San Francisco: Harper & Row, 1987.

Fromm, E. *The Art of Loving*. London: Unwin Books, 1972.

Keen, S. *The Passionate Life: Stages of Loving.* San Francisco: Harper & Row, 1983.

Swami Vivekananda. *Karma Yoga and Bhakti Yoga.* New York: Ramakrishna-Vivekananda Center, rev ed., 1982.

DANCING ON THE RAZOR'S EDGE: THE YOGA OF RELATIONSHIP
BY JOHN WELWOOD, PH.D.

Relationship is a powerful, often dizzying dance of polarities— sometimes delightful and seductive, sometimes fierce and combative, sometimes energizing, sometimes exhausting.

The dance begins as soon as we find ourselves attracted to another person. On the one hand, we long to go out to that person, break out of the shell of separateness, expand our boundaries, and meet this being who moves and touches us in ways that we can hardly begin to understand. On the other hand, we also experience fear—going outside ourselves involves giving up something and we find that we are hanging on for dear life to the very separateness we long to overcome.

The dance of relationship always involves such alternations— between coming together and moving apart, taking hold and letting go, yielding and taking the lead, giving ourselves and maintaining our integrity. And it is not an easy dance to learn. Many couples soon lose the rhythm and wind up deadlocked in opposing positions, knowing only how to attack or how to withdraw. Teachers of this art are few, and as the years go by the conventional dance steps we have been taught seem increasingly stiff, outmoded, and constricting. Where, we may wonder, can we learn to dance with grace and power?

Meditation can teach us a great deal about this dance because it is designed to help us overcome the split between self and other. I am specifically referring here to mindfulness meditation, a formless style of meditation in which one simply sits and follows the breath, allowing thoughts and feelings to arise and pass away. Since this practice provides no fixed object of attention, it allows us to simply be with ourselves and to discover the obstacles we create to avoid being present— such as identifying ourselves with thoughts and feelings we like, while trying to get rid of thoughts and feelings we don't like.

However, if we can come back to the breath and unhook ourselves from identifying with any side in this struggle, we can glimpse a larger,

Feeling is the very root and ground of our existence as conscious entities. And this feeling is joyousness (ananda); to live and to be is joy; suffering is only when we are not able to live and to be as we would.

J. C. CHATTERJI

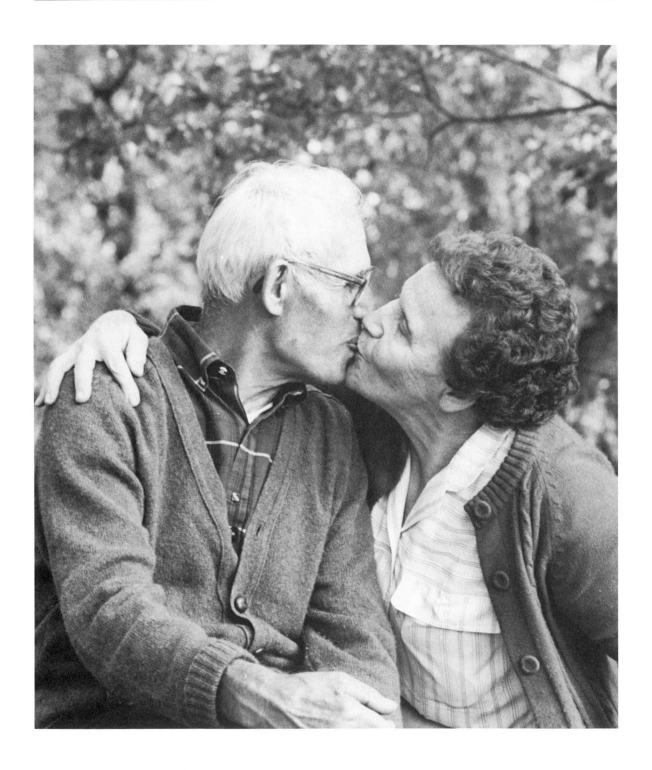

underlying awareness that is free of struggle. These glimpses of our larger nature are like a refreshing breeze. They allow us to relax, to just be here as we are, and to make friends with ourselves.

This style of meditation is a way of working with the basic polarities of being human—polarities that all relationships intensify. On the one hand, it involves settling down on one spot, rooting ourselves to this piece of earth. Coming down to earth, we find that we cannot escape this form, this body, these needs and feelings, this karma, these personal characteristics and traits, this history. Sitting makes a connection with the earth through a balanced, grounded posture—a straight back, neither too tight nor too loose, with upright head and shoulders. On the other hand, following the breath and returning again and again to the present moment allows us to experience a greater sense of openness and space. In this openness we can glimpse a way out of imprisonment in our karma.

In Chinese philosophy these two sides of human nature are called heaven and earth. The heaven principle involves expansiveness and openness. The earth principle involves solidity and groundedness. Maintaining a grounded, upright posture opens up the soft, vulnerable front of the body, through which we let the world and other people in.

We learn from meditation that holding our seat—not getting thrown or carried off by the wild horse of the mind and the emotions—allows us to let go and open out to the world and to others. In a relationship, holding our seat might mean not letting others manipulate or dominate us, but rather maintaining our own vital integrity and power. At the same time, letting go and dissolving back into the breath corresponds in a relationship to not making our personal identity a solid fortress, but being willing to open our heart, let down our guard, and risk ourselves in love. The Buddha likened meditation practice to tuning a musical instrument—the strings must be neither too tight nor too loose. If we hold on too tight, or if we let ourselves go too much, we lose our balance.

In relationship this same kind of balancing act takes place. Somehow we have to respect our own needs and wants (the earth principle) yet also be able to step back from being overly identified with them (the heaven principle). We have to dissolve our boundaries in order to unite with another person, yet if we simply merge with the other, we may lose ourselves in the relationship—which usually spells disaster. Relationship is full of these contradictions.

We want to be free, yet we also want some stability and commitment. How can we have both? We want to be loving, yet a lot of anger

Though on one side we say that the body is perishable and transitory, it is also a Divine manifestation, and could be a source of joy. Each body is a universe, as good a universe as you could conceive.

SWAMI AMAR JYOTI

187

and critical feelings arise. How do we deal with that? How can we surrender in a relationship without losing our power and being controlled by the other person? How can we move close and really get to know the other while continuing to see him or her with fresh eyes? If we could just maintain a safe distance and a clear set of boundaries to protect us from risking too much. . . . Or if we could simply merge with the other person and lose ourselves in the relationship. . . . But neither way alone is satisfactory. In learning to balance between too tight and too loose, our movements become more fluid, and the dance develops grace and vigor.

The path of working with the polarities and contradictions of being human—called in classical Buddhist terms "the middle way"—involves learning not to identify with anything: neither this nor that, neither pleasure nor depression, neither separateness nor togetherness, neither attachment nor detachment. In the practice of the middle way, we are continually coming back to the present, putting aside our attachment to this or that position and seeing just what needs to be done right now. Not that we should never take a stand—right now my relationship with my partner may require me to take a stand, assert what I want, even fight for it if I have to. But tomorrow circumstances may call on me to let go of this stand, give in, and let her needs take precedence.

Hardening into a position, no matter how just it may seem, dulls our sensitivity to what is needed right now and therefore makes us less available to the call of love, less attuned to the rhythm of the dance. The paradox of relationship is that it calls on us to be ourselves fully, to express who we are without hesitation, to take a stand on this earth, and also to let go of our fixed positions and not get solidly identified with them.

Nonattachment in relationship doesn't mean that we should have no needs or that we should pay no attention to them. If we don't respect and acknowledge our real needs, we are not being ourselves, and therefore we have less to offer our partner. Nonattachment in the best sense means that we are not completely identified with our needs, our likes and dislikes. We recognize our needs, yet we can also tap into a larger way of being, a larger awareness inside us where those needs do not have an absolute hold on us. Then we can either assert our desire or let it go, according to the dictates of the moment. When two people become too identified with their positions, they become polarized (for example, "I want more closeness" *vs.* "I want more space"), and the dance grinds to a halt.

We must assume that self-centered consciousness is only a stage, and that some evolutionary process is at work, beyond human design, selecting the whole-centered from the self-centered, empowering the former and disempowering the latter. In fact, evolution could be defined as a process of selection of ever more conscious individuals.

BARBARA MARX HUBBARD

Tantric Buddhism speaks about the middle way as "the razor's edge." If we slip and fall into a solid identification with any position—wanting more closeness or space, separateness or togetherness, freedom or commitment—we do damage to ourselves because we give precedence to the isolated part of us at the expense of the whole of what we are. In order to maintain our balance, we need to keep coming back again and again to the present moment, which is sharp and thin as a razor's edge.

This dynamic balance—continually coming back to now—involves a slight jolt which wakes us up from our fantasies and daydreams. These little moments of waking up to the present—what Shunryu Suzuki Roshi calls "beginner's mind"—are pulsing with uncertainty. In the split second of nowness I realize that I really don't know what's going on. How could I? I just got here! When I return from the fantasy of the relationship I'm in and look into my partner's eyes, I suddenly realize, "I don't know who you are." And further, I don't know who I am, I don't know what this relationship is. In this moment we have the freedom to start fresh again. We don't have to get stuck in our hopes or images about who we are or where this relationship is going. Nor can we make not knowing into a solid position, never making up our minds whether or not to commit ourselves to this partnership—for that too would throw the relationship out of balance.

Dancing on the razor's edge means including and embracing all of what we are as human beings. After a fight with my partner, part of me wants to nurse my anger, and another part of me wants to drop it and express my love instead. This uncertainty brings me back again to the knife edge of the present. Feeling all that I experience at this moment— I am very angry, and I also love you intensely—is quite painful. Yet we can taste in such moments what it means to be human: we have these emotions, yet we do not have to deny or transcend them. Nor do we need to indulge in our angry thoughts, making them into a solid story with which to justify ourselves and attack the other person. Here on this edge of uncertainty, where we cannot settle into this or that position, we have to simply be here and respond to what is happening. The pain of feeling all that we are, stretching to include it all, and not settling into a secure position actually awakens the heart and allows a larger love to flow, free of attachment to any viewpoint.

Personally I have found meditation to be the most effective practice for learning how to face the difficulties of relationship—practice for the further practice of loving another. I don't know which practice is harder.

As a student progresses on the path, he arrives at a highly sensitized condition when dealing with the world, and this becomes painful at times. The problems which thus arise cannot be eliminated, for increasing sensitivity is a natural result of finer mental and emotional development. However, the reaction to difficulties caused by this can be controlled.

PAUL BRUNTON

Building the "Sacred Vessel" of Relationship
by Karen Turner

We who stand are the only animals capable of loving.

Stanley Keleman

At this critical juncture in the evolution of planetary consciousness, we are all being called upon to transform our relationships—from the most intimate to the most casual—into sacred vessels that can be filled with the ever-renewing life of the spirit.

Of course, the embarrassing truth is that we are all quite self-centered and that we spend a great deal of time trying to control one another so we can get what we want. But rather than berating ourselves for this, let us admit it first in the privacy of our own hearts—and then we can set about the alchemical work of transforming the lead of that ego, the lead of our attachments, into the gold of love and surrender.

Certainly we all would agree that there is a force or power at work in the world that is greater than our egos. By viewing our intimate relationships—with our lover or mate, with our friends, with our children, with our parents, and most of all with ourselves—as sacred vessels, sacred opportunities, we can surrender our attachments and our preconceptions to this higher power and learn to love and let go just a little bit more each day. As we do this, we create more consciousness in our personal lives and so contribute to the collective consciousness of our planet.

Another analogy I like to use is that in intimate relationships we have an opportunity to use "muscles" we have not used in a long time—the muscles of letting go and accepting and opening and loving. As we exercise those muscles more and more each day, we contribute to our ability to exercise these qualities in every area of our lives.

To create sacred vessels of our relationships, we must first make clear our intention to live and relate in this way. Openness is required—to other people and to the opportunities for growth inherent in each new situation. Trust is also necessary—in ourselves, one another, and our capacity for self-realization. And so, too, is commitment—commitment to maintaining and nurturing this vessel and to engaging together in the process of transformation. Without these three qualities—openness, trust, and commitment—which form the walls of the sacred vessel, the vessel will not be strong enough to hold the deeply transformative work we must do.

Once the vessel has been forged, the following principles can serve as guidelines on the spiritual path of relationship.

1. **Practice telling and hearing the truth.** We fear the truth because we are afraid of being abandoned or rejected. We do not often consider the

enormous pain we cause to ourselves and others when we don't tell the truth. Set aside some time each week to be completely truthful with each other—even to divulge truths that are very difficult to share. Total honesty can have a cleansing and healing effect on a relationship.

2. Stay with the experience of the present moment. To the best of our ability and with compassion for our limitations, we need to penetrate more and more deeply into our present experience, whether pleasurable or painful. This fidelity to our experience, rather than to some intellectual understanding, can take us beyond simply knowing (which is an ego event) into the eternal now of not knowing, the eternal mystery of Being itself.

With love as a companion we are invincible.

DIANA SALTOON

3. Choose the relationship exactly as it is. By choosing in this way, we take responsibility for our lives and empower ourselves to be active participants in life, rather than victims of or aggressors against life. Taking responsibility keeps us from blaming one another and opens us to the opportunities for growth and learning inherent in our present life situation.

4. Respect, appreciate, and acknowledge yourself and others. Self-respect and respect for others involves a willingness to be open and not fixate on any set of reactions or preconceptions. By deeply honoring, acknowledging, and appreciating our own and each other's uniqueness and wholeness, we set one another free to be who we really are, beyond all the images fabricated by our minds.

5. Recognize your own reflection in the other. We tend to project onto others the parts of ourselves, both positive and negative, that we do not accept in ourselves. Each time we re-own another of these projections, we become a little more aware of our wholeness, and a little less apt to blame another, thus avoiding having to deal with our own emptiness.

6. Share both your grief and your highest visions together. Because of our cultural conditioning, we often find it more difficult to share our highest aspirations and visions than to share our deepest despair. These areas in us are often so precious that we feel extremely vulnerable sharing them. But we need to support one another in responding to a higher, spiritual calling; we need to come to know and trust the light in each other's hearts.

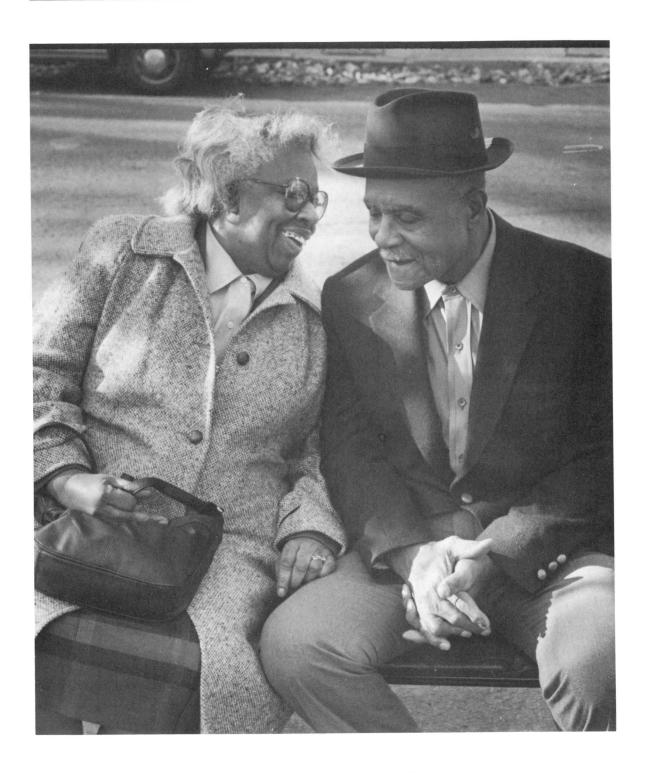

7. Risk being impeccably true to yourself. We often impose form on relationships because we are insecure and afraid of the future. If we allow a relationship to grow naturally, as an expression of our authenticity, an organic form will emerge. Because of our jealousy and insecurity, we try to get others to take care of us, to rescue us from our pain. But it is only by deeply feeling our own pain and grief that we can open our hearts to the suffering of others. Instead of being rescued or cared for, we can actually turn for nurture to the sources of life within and can live from the knowledge that we are each whole unto ourselves and already one with that source.

8. Practice forgiveness. We can facilitate our own and each other's release from suffering by practicing forgiveness. First spend time looking into your own heart to find there the willingness to forgive, and then forgive yourself and others and ask for forgiveness in return. Forgiveness also involves asking ourselves whether we are willing to support each other in becoming whole, no matter how it may affect the form of the relationship.

9. Share your joy, laughter, and playfulness together. Spend time *not* working on the relationship. Paradoxically, as we share our joy, we become more aware of how attached we are to suffering—and can start to let go of that attachment as well.

10. Meditate together. Schedule quiet time, time to "go inside" and share what you find there. Also, *A Course in Miracles* advises us to "remember home" together, to share our deepest longings to return to our true home. This longing, the Course teaches, lies behind the addictions—to food, sex, people, ideas—to which so many of us are prone.

11. Honor separate as well as shared interests, friends, and practices. We need both times of separation and times of union to realize our wholeness. Paradoxically, we can only become one people, one planet, by becoming one, whole, and free within ourselves. Only by first discovering what we want in our personal lives can we come to know that our deepest wish is to become one with God.

12. Explore the relationship of sexuality to spirituality. We need to look carefully at our attitudes toward sexuality. Do we use it to become more aware of our wholeness? Or do we use it to control each other out

Magic strength is hidden in Love. It is the key which opens everything that is closed.

BEINSA DOUNO
(PETER DEUNOV)

of fear and insecurity? Are we consciously choosing to use our sexual energy, our life energy, for spiritual growth? As we turn our relationships into sacred vessels, all the energy generated there can be used to fuel the process of transformation.

13. Get outside help when needed. Many of us tend to idealize our spiritual practice and so do not seek outside help when problems arise in our intimate relationships. But outside input, especially from one who is not caught up in our "couple" system, can help us cut through unconscious and unhealthy patterns and attitudes.

14. Personal relationships reflect global relationships. Together we create the collective consciousness of this planet. What happens to one of us happens, at some level, to us all. By recognizing and sharing our experiences as we attempt to make of our relationships a spiritual path, we can increase our shared awareness of the ways in which we are responsible to ourselves, each other, and the whole earth.

Using these guiding principles, we can begin to make of our intimate relationships a spiritual practice. Day by day, we can learn to be more supportive of each other, more compassionate, more loving, more authentic. The personal, the global, and the transpersonal realms are no longer separate, and the work we do in our personal lives has a significant impact on the lives of billions of people we will never meet.

We all want the same things for ourselves—to love (and be loved), to accept (and be accepted), to forgive (and be forgiven), to serve (and be served). We are one people, nourished by one planet, sustained by one spirit—and the more we can remember this, the more we can "remember home" together and make of this world a sanctuary and a vessel of peace.

UNCONDITIONAL LOVE
BY KEN KEYES, JR.

An example of unconditional love is a mother's love for her young child. She can love her child when he comes into the house covered with mud and tracks it over the recently mopped floor. She can love him when he jumps on the couch after she has told him to clean up in the bathtub. And she can even love him when he yells, "No! I won't!" and she has to

Unconditional love is not blind love, that is, love that fails to recognize differences. On the contrary, unconditional love consciously recognizes the differences.

HAL ZINA BENNETT

Life without love has no meaning. Such a life is a chain of suffering, of successive fallings and risings.

BEINSA DOUNO
(PETER DEUNOV)

pick him up and carry him into the bathroom while he's kicking and screaming.

She's completely opposed to his behavior and doesn't like that at all. And yet she still loves him. She doesn't confuse the tape player with the tape that is being played out!

It is often easiest for us to love very young children unconditionally. They are such tiny bundles of cuddly, soft cuteness that pull on our heartstrings. It is a much greater challenge to apply this to our relationship partner. The multifaceted involvement of living together brings out demanding programming we never knew we had!

Yet if we learn to recognize the programs we don't like as just mental habits we picked up, we can learn to go beyond them and love unconditionally.

What keeps me going is the knowledge that the world was created to express love and as an expression of love.

BERNIE SIEGEL

SACRED SEXUALITY
BY GEORG FEUERSTEIN, PH.D.

Sacred sexuality is the art and discipline of turning love-making into whole-body loving, of experiencing ourselves and our partner against the eternal backdrop of unconditional love (prema) or bliss (ananda) of the ultimate Reality. In other words, sacred sexuality is the exercise of our sexual faculties in the context of a spiritually committed life. It is based on the view that the sexual force is precious and sacred and not to be squandered.

So long as we look upon our partner as a "meat body," we are apt to treat him or her as a means to an end—a tool for gratifying our own pleasure. Sacred sexuality, by contrast, presupposes that we are capable of seeing ourselves and our partner in the light of the Divine. It presupposes that we are able to encounter the spiritual Reality, or transcendental Self, in our sexual relationship and play. Only then can we go beyond the anxious pursuit of orgasm. We must bring to our sexual relationship a measure of self-transcendence (surrender) and relaxation of the need to be merely pleasurized.

Orgasm is the closest simulation of the absolute bliss (ananda) that, according to the Hindu tradition, we are all unconsciously striving for. But orgasmic pleasure is only a trickle in comparison to that bliss, and it is of course disappointingly ephemeral. The nervous discharge that accompanies orgasm creates a momentary state of balance, but that balance is on a very reduced level of energy.

When sex is an expression of love, . . . the emotion experienced at the moment of orgasm is not hostility or triumph, but union with the other person.

ROLLO MAY

The practitioners of Tantrism, or Tantra, recognize the error in this popular approach, which seeks self-completion by external means, namely sexual union. They are more interested in heightening the level of psychosomatic energy and in intensifying awareness, until there is the breakthrough into the transcendental dimension of bliss. They engage sexual intercourse as a spiritual discipline rather than for hedonistic reasons.

This approach entails the insight that every individual is, psychologically speaking, both male and female, and that therefore the desired unitive or balanced state does not occur externally but internally, in consciousness. Thus, for the Tantric practitioner, the outward sexual act is essentially a symbolic ritual of the real work, which is performed in consciousness. Indeed, the "right-handed" schools of Tantrism do not even condone actual sexual congress.

However, the "left-handed" approach, which involves sexual intercourse (*maithuna*) with a suitable partner, has the advantage of increasing the level of psychosomatic energy and thus of including the physical dimension in the process of psychospiritual transformation. Actual sexual intercourse involves an energy exchange between the partners in the Tantric ritual, which enhances the unification process that is strived for on the level of consciousness.

At the point of enlightenment, the Tantric practitioner realizes the transcendental unity of male and female, Shiva and Shakti. This condition is known as "great delight" (maha-sukha), since it cannot be diminished by anything, not even by the act of ejaculation, which typically concludes the male partner's experience of sexual pleasure in ordinary circumstances.

Tantra is the technology of joy on many levels—from sexual pleasure to transcendental bliss. It is a yogic art that explores the hidden dimensions of the unity of body and mind, which modern science is only now beginning to acknowledge. It reminds us that our guilt about sex is only an added complication that we superimpose on our false relationship to sexual pleasure.

Instead of viewing sex as a means of higher human growth, we tend to use it as a fleeting consolation or a way of asserting power and dominance over another. Perhaps our guilt feelings are not so much about engaging our "lower" functions as about not finding the bliss of transcendental consciousness.

Tantrism challenges us to a radically different view about ourselves and sexuality: to view sex as a lawful, if limited, expression of our in-

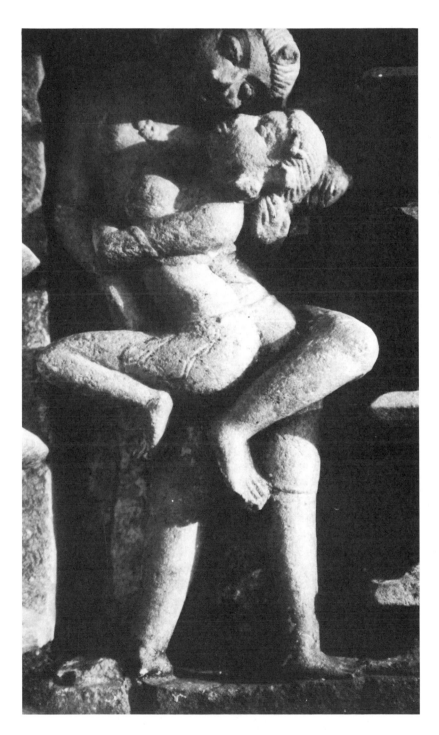

*Love contains everything, and
outside of love is a void and
everlasting nothingness.*

OMRAAM MIKHAEL
AIVANHOV

nate bliss, and at the same time as a means of getting in touch with that unalloyed delight that is the very nature of reality. According to Tantrism, the body is the temple of the divine or transcendental reality. But for this to be functionally true of us, and not merely in principle true, we must discover and live from the point of view of that great delight. Then everything, including our sexuality, will be transformed. Our lives become creative play.

When we as Westerners practice sacred sexuality, we must first of all avoid becoming neurotic about orgasm—either having it or not having it. Rather, we should relax our concern about it and instead find the delight that comes with being simply present and in heartfelt relationship with one another. This also entails that we should not indulge in erotic fantasies about our partner but actually see him or her. Without seeing or experiencing our partner as he or she is, we cannot be drawn into the great Mystery that lies beyond the masks we habitually wear in order to defend ourselves. Fantasies prevent us from being real and present in the moment. They block out the Mystery of life and exclude us from its innate bliss.

Sacred sexuality is a meditative occasion. Hence we should prepare for it as we would for meditation. This includes, for instance, consecrating our bedroom by tidying it and, perhaps, burning incense and decorating it with flowers. We should also arrange to be undisturbed for a few hours. Some couples keep their bedroom very tidy, clean, and "conscious" at all times, which is preferable. Long-time practitioners often decorate it with spiritual art, reminding them of the higher purpose of sex—Tibetan thankas, paintings, posters, sculptures, gongs. Or they have a picture of their teacher prominently displayed. Some couples develop their own elaborate ritual, complete with the recitation of potent sounds (mantra), the drawing of mystic diagrams (yantra), and similar yogic ceremonial aids. Others like to keep it very simple.

What is most important, however, is always to bring the right attitude to the occasion. Whether we are in a mood of sobriety or gaiety, we should always remain aware of the sacredness of the sexual play. Obviously, it is advisable to engage sex only when we feel well, balanced, and positive and to abstain when we are sick, agitated, collapsed, or needy. In other words, we should approach the sexual occasion as much as possible in a condition of wholeness, rather than expecting to be made whole or to be consoled or fulfilled by it. Then sacred sex will help integrate our being on a deeper level.

Part of preparing our personal environment for the sacred occasion

Our deepest, most committed and responsible love—the love we experience for life, for others, for ourselves; the love that stirs us to find meaning in humble things—flows primarily from our fully developed, autonomous self.

MARSHA SINETAR

is that we cleanse our body and mind. To shake off the concerns of the day, we would do well to relax or sit in meditation for a while, preceded by a shower or bath and followed, perhaps, by a gentle mutual massage.

The actual sexual play is entirely a matter of personal style and preference. Whether we are active/performative or more passive/contemplative, our attention should be on being present here and now, feeling our body-mind and that of our partner, and cultivating the great eloquent Silence as it is expanding in us.

In Tantrism, the woman generally sits in the man's lap, which means that she is in control of all movement. Taoism permits a great variety of postures. It also recommends all kinds of fairly technical tricks for intensifying the build-up of nervous energy during sex play. In the last analysis, however, it is not so important what we do. What matters is how we do what we do. It is our inner disposition that is critical. This cannot be emphasized enough.

Clearly, the right attitude to sacred sex cannot be cultivated in isolation from our behavior during the rest of the day. We cannot hope to embrace our partner with love and reverence at night but treat her or him as a casual sex object during the day. The success of our sexual discipline depends on our attitude to life as a whole. We cannot compartmentalize our existence without damaging our psyche and relationships.

For the duration of sacred sex, the Tantric partners look upon each other as god and goddess. Their awareness of each other is transplanted from the material level to the domain of energy and beyond. For most of us who have very little background in visualization and religious mythology, this will not be possible at first or as a rule. However, we can all develop the ability to approach our sexual partner with reverence and clarity and in a mood of love and surrender.

Gradually we will be able to see more in him or her than the individual who is so familiar to us. In fact, we will find that he or she becomes less and less familiar and more and more part of the great Mystery, which is our hidden essence.

Deep and conscious breathing is the principal means of remaining sensitive to the energy dimension during sexual intercourse. This practice is especially important when we approach orgasm. It permits us to distribute the built-up preorgasmic energy throughout our body, thus preventing orgasm, which generally ends the sacred energy play. However, if orgasm occurs, we should simply remain present in our sensory awareness and also in our love-communion, using the breath to guide the mounting sensation to the body as a whole (rather than merely to

A free heart is a heart delivered from the gusts and storms of the affections and passions; the assailing touch of grief, wrath, hatred, fear, inequality of love, trouble of joy, pain of sorrow fall away from the equal heart, and leave it a thing large, calm, equal, luminous, divine.

SRI AUROBINDO

199

the genitals) and, beyond the body, to our partner and the cosmos.

It is important not to disengage physical contact abruptly. Intercourse is an intense mingling of our energies, particularly when it is combined with conscious discipline. If orgasm is avoided, our body will remain highly charged after intercourse. However, it is unwise to manipulate our nervous system to the point of near-orgasm if we cannot live with the resulting charge afterward without becoming frustrated. Again, breathing can be very useful in removing possible tension resulting from overstimulation without orgasmic discharge.

Couples interested in sacred sex must be willing to experiment and make mistakes. This is not a path for the meek, the weak, or the indiscriminate. It is very easy to delude onself. Therefore it is always good to remember that, at least according to Tantrism, the ultimate form of sexual congress does not involve any sexual excitation whatsoever. The couple experience themselves as male god (Shiva) and goddess (Shakti), absorbed in bliss rather than orgasm.

Thus, the Tantric yogi or yogini sacrifices orgasm for the great bliss of Self-realization. Western practitioners of the art of sacred sexuality should, however, be wary of pursuing that bliss as they might pursue a pet idea or favored activity. It escapes us even as we make it our goal, because it is ever present. Our primary obligation is, therefore, to be present and to discover that bliss in every moment, whether we are engaging in sex or not.

Sacred sex is simply a temporary intensification of our general commitment to a self-transcending life. Sex is never our salvation. It is only another, if powerful, opportunity to realize the great Tantric truth that we are presently free and inherently blissful.

RESOURCES

Books

Aivanhov, O. M. *Love and Sexuality*. Frejus, France: Prosveta, 1988. 2 vols. Distributed by Prosveta U.S.A., Los Angeles.

Anand, M. *The Art of Sexual Ecstasy: The Path of Sacred Sexuality for Western Lovers*. Los Angeles: J. P. Tarcher, 1989.

Douglas, N., and P. Slinger. *Sexual Secrets: The Alchemy of Ecstasy*. Rochester, VT: Destiny Books, 1979.

Feuerstein, G. *Sacred Sexuality: Living the Vision of the Erotic Spirit*. Los Angeles: J. P. Tarcher, 1992.

Orgasm is the quintessential paradox and, perhaps because of it, the quintessential pleasure in the entire range of human experience.

THOMAS SZASZ

————, ed. *Enlightened Sexuality: Essays on Body-Positive Spirituality*. Freedom, CA: Crossing Press, 1989.

Henderson, J. *The Lover Within: Opening to Energy in Sexual Practice*. Barrytown, NY: Station Hill Press, 1987.

Meldman, L. W. *Mystical Sex: Love, Ecstasy, and the Mystical Experience*. Tucson, AZ: Harbinger House, 1990.

Welwood, J., ed. *Challenge of the Heart: Love, Sex, and Intimacy*. Boston, MA: Shambhala Publications, 1985.

————. *Journey of the Heart: Intimate Relationship and the Path of Love*. New York: HarperCollins, 1990.

Periodicals

Ecstasy: The Journal of Divine Eroticism. A quarterly magazine dedicated to promoting the awareness that sexuality is inherently sacred. P.O. Box 862, Ojai, CA 93024.

Tantra: The Magazine. A quarterly publication that seeks to make Tantric ideas and practices accessible to Western readers. P.O. Box 79, Torreon, NM 87061.

Love as a personal path involves plowing the coarse and rocky ground of ego, breaking up the hardened places inside us, refining and enriching this soil so that life can grow more abundantly in us.

JOHN WELWOOD

TANTRIC CELIBACY AND THE MYSTERY OF EROS
BY STUART SOVATSKY, PH.D.

The terrain of conventional sexuality has been well charted over the past twenty years. Yet there are very few maps of that little-understood territory known as *brahmacarya*, or yogic celibacy. Some might think it a desert or a lonely island, others an earthly impossibility. Nevertheless, just about all of us find ourselves celibate, whether by choice or by circumstance, for at least some time during our lives. And periods of celibacy may be becoming more commonplace and prolonged these days, as our culture swings away from the freewheeling sexuality of the '60s toward a more thoughtful and discriminating attitude toward relationship. Here I hope to show that, like conventional sexuality, yogic celibacy offers much to those willing to experiment with its age-old methods.

On the basis of extensive personal experience and interviews with other practitioners, I have discovered that the brahmacarya lifestyle actually has much in common with conventional sexuality. Both are erotic, both are problematic at times, yet both are filled with life-enhancing potential. Any discussion that polarizes celibacy and sexuality distracts

Caring for other people tends to produce a joy in their good that lifts us beyond everyday needs and desires. Loving service and friendship . . . have a tendency toward metanormal delight.

MICHAEL MURPHY

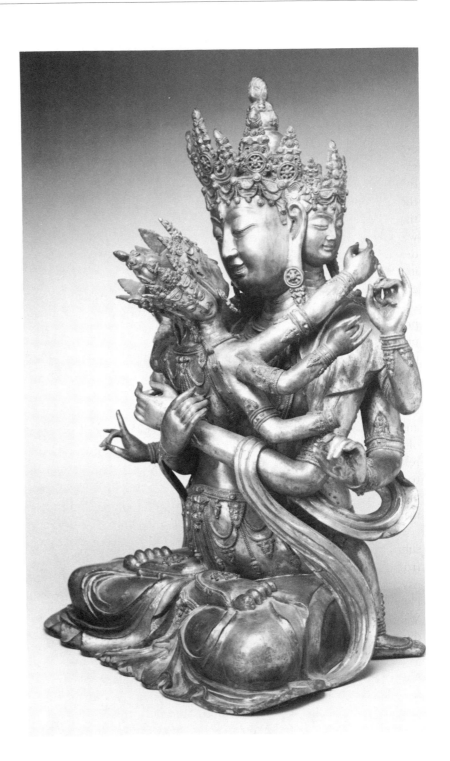

us from such deeper questions as, What exactly is eros? and, What is erotic and sexual liberation? That is, how can we act upon erotic feelings in a way that secures our greatest growth, intimacy, and pleasure?

Is it possible that such feelings may in fact signal an opportune time to meditate? Or that perhaps they occur to be enjoyed in themselves, just as they are? What would happen to one who repeatedly interpreted erotic sensations in these ways? Although we have been taught that such a person would become painfully repressed, there are other views on the matter. The great Indian saint Ramakrishna, for example, noted that the penultimate celibate state in yoga "was one in which it seemed that all the pores of the skin were like female organs, and intercourse was taking place over the whole body."[1] In light of such an authoritative description, the sex/celibacy debate loses its potency. Rather than trying to prove which life-style is better or more correct, let us approach erotic feelings with "beginner's mind," i.e., without preconceptions.

Curiously, beginner's mind is also the central attitude behind the practice of brahmacarya. This Sanskrit word means literally "one who practices" (acarya) the way of the Absolute (brahman). Whether explicitly or implicitly, the true brahmacarin is asking the question, What is the essential erotic life when we are free of accumulated concepts, habits, and social conditionings? Is it, as Wilhelm Reich and other Western theorists maintain, a system of physiological responses, emotions, and behaviors that inevitably lead to genital orgasm? Or is this just one of numerous possible ways of embodying eros in ourselves and our love relationships? In this age of sexual sophistication, it may sound strange to pretend that we don't really know all that "erotic feelings" may signify. But it is precisely through such an innocent attitude that the brahmacarin hopes to make some truly new discoveries about sexuality.

The yogic model of the individual constitution, with its various subtle bodies, allows for a natural process of energetic transmutation from the physical to the spiritual levels of our being. Modern Western psychosexual theory does not include such a continuum, nor does it include processes of transmutation. According to Alexander Lowen and Wilhelm Reich, two of the originators of the psychosexual model, individual growth takes place within a closed system whose energetic transformations require frequent discharge in genital orgasm.

> When growth has reached its natural limits, some other use
> must be made of the excess energy that is being produced. . . .
> In the higher animals, the excess energy is discharged in the

As you allow the Beloved to grow within you, you will discover a steadfastness to the spiritual journey that comes your way in the most remarkable fashion.

JEAN HOUSTON

sexual function, as Wilhelm Reich showed.

Maturity means that the energy that was formerly needed for the growth process is now available for discharge.[2]

According to yogic physiology, by contrast, this excess energy is actually sublimated as part of an eight-step, month-long transformation of food into bodily tissues and finally into light energy. In the seventh and eighth steps, physical sexual essence (bindu) sublimates to subtle light-consciousness energy (ojas), thereby creating a spiritual force (virya).[3] More than one sexual release per month is considered a kind of "over-harvesting," which disrupts the eighth step and depletes the individual of ojas.

We can think of this process as a bodily ecology of sexual energy, with its own cyclical rhythms. Ojas, which can be thought of as a powerful alchemical distillate of the hormones of sexual motivation, helps nourish maturation and growth processes in ways not envisioned by Lowen or Reich. Herein lies the yogic basis for the sexual life-style of brahmacarya; it is not a moralistic repression, but a uniquely pleasurable process of sexual transmutation in which the practices of yoga are fueled by high-octane ojas. As one of my research subjects noted, "It is really quite hedonistic, only of another sort. Otherwise, I wouldn't be doing it."

From the outside, brahmacarya may appear to be asexual. Yet internally one feels permeated with eros, what mystics have called the "inward caresses of the divine." Ordinary life activities like breathing and moving reveal a previously hidden, pleasurable warmth. A pervasive, sensual, yet non-grasping intimacy with the world slowly melts egoic isolation. What was once taken to be simply and obviously sex now emerges as intricately complex and mysterious. The familiar truths about sex and conventional routes of sexual expression begin to appear as one largely overworked possibility among many. The erotic sense of one's own body, one's attractiveness to others, and the meaning of gender, orgasm, and psychosexual development can no longer be explained with prevailing concepts and theories. But it becomes very clear how sexual energy is both a basis for pleasurable sensation and a maturational force.

In fact, one has the sense that the body is undergoing another kind of puberty, resulting in a transformation on a par with adolescence in terms of gender identity, bodily capacities, and sexual understanding. In other words, a whole new erotic universe emerges. Ken Wilber alludes to this "post-genital" sexuality when he states that the maintenance of

A truly philosophic attitude is neither ascetic nor hedonistic. It takes what is worthy from both—not by arithmetical computation to arrive at equal balance but by wise insight to arrive at harmonious living.

PAUL BRUNTON

the genital stage of development "beyond its normal and necessary development period represents the refusal to accept its death and discover higher states of whole-body ecstasy, ecstasy beyond the genitals."[4]

Not that the pleasures of brahmacarya are easily won, the change-over of erotic meanings and body energetics, especially in our hypersexualized culture, requires a steadfast discipline and a sensitive appreciation for subtle, incremental changes. Sexual desire, in fact, often increases during brahmacarya—a sign, paradoxically, that transmutation is taking place. Obviously, this may also create inner struggles, for the advanced brahmacarin as well as for the beginner. But even a conventional sexual life-style confronts one with problems, and brahmacarins must learn to accept and work with any issues that arise.

They must discover ways of expressing these heightened feelings of love and attraction that are consistent with their brahmacarya sexuality. They must watch for the ego's attempts at "spiritual materialism"—i.e., the tendency to use spiritual practice to feel superior to others. At the same time, they must maintain the regime of yoga practices and pure diet needed to assist in rechanneling the energy "up and in," rather than "down and out." Above all, brahmacarins must keep a positive and accepting attitude toward sexual feelings. Otherwise, repression may very possibly occur.

The contempoary notion of sexual liberation interprets erotic sensations in terms of the primacy of the genital orgasm. Thus, sexual liberation has come to mean freeing oneself from externally imposed restrictions on having sex. Through brahmacarya one can step back from this hundred-year-long experiment in sexual liberation and approach the matter with the innocence of "not knowing." The erotic world that emerges may reveal that, after all is said and done, the experienced mystery of eros, of love-attraction, of procreation, birth, and rebirth, and of individual psychosexual unfoldment is deeper and more subtle than the words of any theory can describe. And, as we in the West learn more about yogic understandings of psychosexual development, we might humbly admit that we are just beginning to fathom the full expanse of the erotic universe.

Love pulls man's straining world together; love carries man beyond the constrictions of culture.

ERNEST BECKER

RESOURCES

Books

Brown, G. *The New Celibacy: A Journey to Love, Intimacy, and Good Health in a New Age.* New York: McGraw-Hill, 1989.

Ranke-Heinemann, U. *Eunuchs for the Kingdom of Heaven: Women, Sexuality, and the Catholic Church*. New York: Doubleday, 1990.

Sovatsky, S. *Passions of Innocence: Tantric Celibacy and the Mysteries of Eros*. Rochester, VT: Inner Traditions, 1992.

Thomas, G. *Desire and Denial: Celibacy and the Church*. Boston, MA: Little, Brown & Co., 1986.

Notes

[1] E. Dimock, *The Place of the Hidden Moon* (Chicago: University of Chicago Press, 1966), p. 4.

[2] Alexander Lowen, *Love and Orgasm* (New York: New American Library, 1967), p. 57.

[3] Ravi Dass and Aparna, *The Marriage and Family Book* (New York: Schocken, 1978), p. 66; and Sri Aurobindo and the Mother, *On Love* (Pondicherry, India: Sri Aurobindo Ashram, 1973).

[4] K. Wilber, *Up from Eden* (Garden City, NY: Anchor/Doubleday, 1981), p. 213.

PART FOUR

THE PATH OF WORK: KARMA YOGA

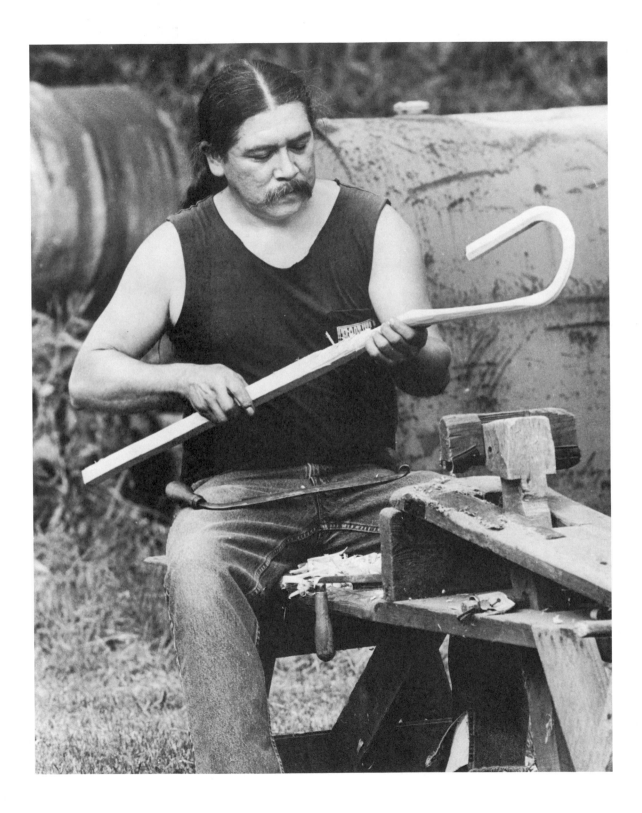

TEN

A Labor of Love

For any spiritual path to be meaningful today, it must be grounded in our everyday experience. In other words, it must take into account that most of us have to work long hours every day in order to procure our livelihood. Well over 2,000 years ago, the yoga tradition came up with an answer that is still relevant today: karma yoga, the path of self-transcending action. This chapter offers perspectives on the pressing issue of how to combine the need for contemplation and inwardness with the need to take care of our material circumstances. Karma yoga has an encouraging message for those who are worried that their busy lives will exclude them from spiritual growth and happiness. It teaches that we need not abandon work. On the contrary, we must embrace it, while at the same time developing a new inner attitude toward it.

Ecstasy lies in details, in what my friend Jack London calls "the yoga of the household."

MORRIS BERMAN

ACTION, INACTION, AND THE TRANSCENDENCE OF ACTION

There are many possible approaches to realizing wholeness and recovering our blissful spiritual identity. Some people are able to summon the critical faculties required for the successful practice of jnana yoga, and a few others have the capacity for the prolonged concentration called for on the path of raja yoga. Then there are those few who are emotionally fluid and mature enough to qualify for bhakti yoga.

However, everyone is active and capable of inspecting the consequences of his or her actions. This is the domain of karma yoga. The Sanskrit word *karma* means "action" or "work." It also refers to the moral consequences of one's actions. Thus morally sound actions lead to morally or spiritually desirable qualities in one's life. Conversely, morally unsound or reprehensible actions lead to moral or spiritual consequences that are negative and detrimental to life. These two types of action and reaction can be summarized as "good karma" and "bad karma."

Yogis, however, endeavor to escape this cycle of action and reaction altogether. Some try to do this by retreating into solitude in remote mountain caves and forests. But even they meditate, eat, drink, and do all the other tasks required to maintain life. Even when we are completely passive, we still must breathe, and breathing is a form of karma, which, according to Hindu metaphysics, is not without moral consequences. In other words, we cannot cease to be active and reap the fruit of our actions. This lesson was taught over two millennia ago by the God-man Krishna, whose teachings are recorded in the *Bhagavad Gita*.

Our only route of escape lies in the way we relate to our actions—in our inner attitude. It is in and through the mind that we can transcend action by shifting our focus of identity from the ego to the Self.

Ordinarily, our actions are infused with our egoic desires and motives. As practitioners of karma yoga, we adopt a different principle of operation: We do what is appropriate, and we do it without selfish attachment. In Swami Vivekananda's words: "Let things work; let the brain centres work; work incessantly, but let not a ripple conquer the mind. Work as if you were a stranger in this land, a sojourner. Work incessantly, but do not bind yourselves."[1]

Our actions cease to be binding when they are rendered as service. Karma yoga thus consists in dedicating all our actions to a higher source. Instead of acting for selfish reasons, we simply practice the art of self-surrender in all our deeds. Such self-surrender is possible when we constantly remember "who" is the true author of all actions. The yogic view is that the myriad processes of life all happen spontaneously, and the ego-personality artificially inserts itself, presuming to be at the center of existence. Nothing could be farther from the truth!

By habitually referring everything to itself, the ego thus piles up karmic baggage that constantly threatens to squash it. Freedom from this burden is possible only when we deflate the ego and recognize its artificial nature. Then we are able to let life flow freely, without clenching our hands into fists and knitting our brows. Our actions will become more and more spontaneous and truly creative, and the original actor of life's drama, the Self, will shine through all our work. Our life becomes service. When asked what is the best way to pay off "bad karma," the woman known as Peace Pilgrim answered in true yogic fashion: by getting busy to serve in any way possible.

For Peace Pilgrim, as for the great spiritual teachers of the East, peace of mind is acquired when work is turned into selfless service. From 1953 until her death in 1981, she walked tens of thousands of miles, traveling throughout the United States on foot to proclaim and demonstrate the eternal values of peace and love.

This illumined karma-yogini saw retirement, which is a big problem for many people in our society, as a unique opportunity to practice self-giving through service. Peace Pilgrim believed that everyone has a calling, which they can discover as they attune themselves to the higher reality. Her life bears out that it is possible, even in our frenetic Western society, to live according to higher principles and find profound peace and joy.

Altruistic, humanitarian activities give deep satisfaction and a sense of fulfilling one's true purpose in life.

ROBERTO ASSAGIOLI

RESOURCES

Books

Dooling, D. M., ed. *A Way of Working: The Spiritual Dimension of Craft.* New York: Parabola Books, 1986.

Feuerstein, G. *The Bhagavad-Gita: Its Philosophy and Cultural Setting.* Wheaton, Il.: Quest Books, 1983.

Peace Pilgrim: Her Life and Work in Her Own Words. Santa Fe, NM: Ocean Tree Books, 1992.

Welwood, J. *Ordinary Magic: Everyday Life as Spiritual Path.* Boston: Shambhala, 1992.

Periodicals

Friends of Peace Pilgrim newsletter, published by the non-profit organization of the same name, located at 43480 Cedar Avenue, Hemet, CA 92544. Tel. (714) 927-7678. This organization also publishes books and tapes on Peace Pilgrim.

IF YOU DO WHAT YOU LOVE, WILL THE MONEY FOLLOW?
BY D. PATRICK MILLER

Perhaps the foremost prophet of "do what you love" is the woman who wrote the book on the subject: Marsha Sinetar, an organizational psychologist, writer, and former school principal who made her own career

A person who is always under the spell of money can never be just.

DEMOCRITUS

No man is to be judged by the mere nature of his duties, but all should be judged by the manner and the spirit in which they perform them.

SWAMI VIVEKANANDA

change over ten years ago, when she could no longer ignore the "prompting from within" to find a new and more fulfilling way of life.

I happened across Sinetar's book several years ago, when its title caught my eye and pushed one of my most sensitive buttons. As a writer who had struggled for nearly a decade to focus my talent and earn a living from it, I found Sinetar's title unrealistic and galling. But her text, which previews the stages of psychological and spiritual growth along the way to finding fulfilling employment, proved helpful and inspiring. For me, it was the beginning of a more conscious and intensive study of the path to "right livelihood" in twentieth-century capitalist America.

I have come to feel that "do what you love, the money will follow" functions less as a guarantee than as a kind of mantra. I believe it to be a spiritual cue for our times, urging people to begin the daunting task of unifying their personal, political, and spiritual ideals with their work and source of income. In an affluent country where, as Sinetar points out, as much as 95 percent of our working population say they do not enjoy the work they do, it is a radical idea, easily lending itself to ridicule or instant dismissal from skeptics—as well as superficial misinterpretation from many who want it to pay off instantly.

According to Sinetar, there are three common misunderstandings of her message:

1. Desire for a quick answer. "The question I'm always hearing," says Sinetar, "is 'How do I do it? Tell me now; your book didn't tell me exactly.' But the heart of right livelihood is taking the time to do things well, honoring the task, and not worrying so much about the fruits of your labor. This is a very difficult concept for Westerners, because we've been schooled to believe that our worth is connected to our bankroll."

2. Misjudgment of talents. "People often don't realize what their real talents are or don't have enough practical experience in what they want to undertake. The best example is that of the typical writer. It takes a long time to build up the necessary skill, reputation, and track record to make it. But people want to have the money rolling in right away."

3. Not knowing how much is enough. "Some people know what would be good for them to do, but they're ill-prepared for the economic realities of their new profession. A secure, high-paying job may have become thankless—but switching to something that's personally fulfilling while failing to sustain their accustomed life-style can be too much sacrifice for some."

The core of Sinetar's message is that the decision to pursue fulfilling work must have a spiritual, not economic, inspiration. Thus the money "follows" in more ways than one; it cannot serve as a first priority. "Right livelihood implies a long-term commitment that's not necessarily going to be easy," Sinetar cautions. "A weathering and cultivation of the human being takes place over the long haul. Maybe we haven't found the right teacher, maybe we're not being completely honest with ourselves, maybe we just want something for nothing. Letting go of all this is part of our spiritual homework."

Man shall not live by bread alone.

MATTHEW 4:4.

Sinetar also stresses that doing what you love is not necessarily synonymous with doing what you *feel* like doing. "Doing what you love means doing what you respect," she remarks, "doing what's in accord with your highest values, what brings up your self-esteem and elevates you morally. Doing what you feel like doing may mean sleeping late, eating popcorn, and watching TV. Right livelihood implies mastery, and mastery doesn't come by caving in when the going gets tough. It comes from repeating the task, even when it's dull; from working when it's beautiful outside and you'd rather play."

Yet for those who are not sure what their right livelihood might be, Sinetar suggests taking a closer look at the things they do now for recreation. "People who don't know what they really want to do probably haven't looked at what they really enjoy, what engages all their enthusiasm and assertion. People who are active and assertive tend to know what they want. It seems quite possible to me that people who don't know what they would love to do are in a depressed state."

Like the larger path to spiritual maturity of which it is a part, the path to right livelihood has no shortcuts. As much as I have fretted and panicked over the money problem in my own discovery of the work I love, I have to admit that the question of monetary reward pales beside the inner strength that the process of discovery builds. Simply by investigating the *possibility* of doing what you love, you initiate a meditation that, if sustained, can provide far-reaching changes both in your own life and in the life of society.

There is no special trick to keeping the meditation going; it all boils down to honesty, which must be chosen, renewed, and strengthened countless times along the way. However much we may long for a financial rescue from "the daily grind," the only lasting liberation, it seems, derives from one of the simplest of spiritual strategies: the truth will set you free.

RESOURCES

Books

Anderson, N. *Work With Passion: How to Do What You Love for a Living.* Carroll & Graf with Whatever Publishing [now New World Library], 1987.

Dominguez, J., and V. Robin. *Your Money or Your Life.* New York: Viking, 1992.

Needleman, J. *Money and the Meaning of Life.* New York: Doubleday/ Currency Books, 1991.

Phillips, M. *The Seven Laws of Money.* New York: Random House, 1974.

Sinetar, M. *Do What You Love, The Money Will Follow: Discovering Your Right Livelihood.* New York: Dell, 1989.

Cassette

Transforming Your Relationship With Money & Achieving Financial Independence, an audiocassette/workbook course based on the seminar by Joseph R. Dominguez. Available from the New Road Map Foundation, P.O. Box 15981. Seattle, WA 98115.

TAKING MONEY SERIOUSLY
BY JACOB NEEDLEMAN, PH.D.

Money is the principal means by which modern man [and woman] enters into the intense world of desire, fear, pleasure and pain, achievement and failure, sex, friendship, courage, loyalty, deceit, cunning, philosophizing, knowledge-gathering, manufacturing of goods, arts, fun, entertainment, competition—all the impulses and activities that make up this round of life called the world in Western traditions, samsara in Eastern traditions. The other world, the world of the spirit, is approached through the increase of attention in oneself, through consciousness of oneself in the midst of hell. The awareness of hell is the escape from hell, or the beginning of the escape.

The first practical step that an individual can take to free himself from the thrall of money is not to turn away from it, but to take it even

It is usually the moneyless aspirants who decry wealth and praise poverty (calling it simplicity). If money can chain a man more tightly to materialism, it can also give him the conditions whereby he can set to work freeing himself from materialism.

PAUL BRUNTON

Unless a person takes charge of them, both work and free time are likely to be disappointing.

MIHALY CSIKSZENTMIHALYI

more seriously, to study himself with such diligence and concern that the very act of self-study becomes as vivid and intense as the desires and fears he is studying.

Excerpted from J. Needleman, *Money and the Meaning of Life* (New York: Doubleday/Currency Books, 1991), p. 171. By permission of the publisher.

LIFE AS SERVICE: AN INTERVIEW WITH RAM DASS
BY STEPHAN BODIAN

What is your day-to-day practice like?

My primary practice is guru kripa, the method of the guru, which involves maintaining a somewhat continuous dialogue with him. I carry his presence inside me all the time, and I relate to him about every situation.

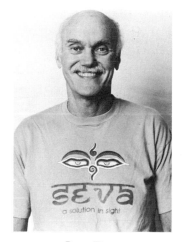

RAM DASS

In addition, Neem Karoli Baba's instructions to me nearly twenty years ago to feed and serve people, and the fact that his lineage in the Hindu tradition is Hanuman [the monkey god who lives only to serve Ram], leads me to constantly be exploring the ways in which service can be the form of bhakti yoga that brings me closer to freedom.

I've always done lots of service, like lecturing, teaching, working with people who are sick or dying, but then I would go meditate in order to cool myself out. I became interested in why I couldn't do the service itself as the vehicle for getting cooled out. Why did I have to rely on dhyana yoga [meditation] rather than karma yoga? Why couldn't karma yoga be complete unto itself? So I decided to throw myself into service as hard as I could. I just kept saying yes: I'm working with AIDS people, I'm working with dying people, I'm teaching courses on aging, I'm doing individual therapy, I help run the Seva Foundation—just more and more stuff, just "yes, yes, yes." And I'm learning where the toxicities are. My sadhana [spiritual practice] now is examining how I get caught in service, how the grabbing starts, where I lose the injunction of the *Bhagavad Gita* that says, "To do pure Dharma, don't identify with the actor or the fruits of action."

You're pushing yourself to an edge, then, in the context of service.

Yes, I always do that. I want to see if it works—and if it doesn't, I want to find out why. I want to see where I have to clean up my act so it will work. I know it's possible because Hanuman did nothing but serve Ram, and he had this incredible energy because of the purity of his service. So I'm just examining my impurities, if you will, discovering where I have to tune up my vehicle.

Where do you draw the line? For example, why sleep? Why eat? Why eat as much as you do? Where does one stop giving out completely and start taking care of oneself? Is there a limit?

Even that distinction—taking care of oneself versus giving to others—is a model that gets in the way. If it's working right, when you're giving out, you're also taking care of yourself. My book *How Can I Help?* focuses on how it works both ways. If it doesn't, something is wrong. Through service you should be getting fed, getting energized, becoming lighter and more spacious.

Of course, all this is theoretical. Part of its works for me and part of it doesn't. What I need to do is to keep zeroing in on the part that doesn't and keep explaining it to myself and to everybody else until we can see why, because I'm sure service can be a pure upaya [method for achieving enlightenment]. I just don't know yet how to articulate it, and I can't find the books that do.

In other words, it's not that there's something wrong with serving so selflessly, but rather that there's something wrong with the vehicle doing the serving that needs to be taken care of.

Exactly. And it's a fascinating adventure for me because I feel I'm getting closer to my lineage, which is Hanuman and Maharaj-ji [Neem Karoli Baba]. Maharaj-ji used to sleep two hours a night. The rest of the time he would be surrounded by people; he would be yelling and teaching and throwing people out and feeding people and doing whatever he did, and maybe he was doing that on other planes in the room as well—I don't know. In Burma we didn't eat after 11 in the morning and I found that I slept much less. The fact that we slept four hours a night didn't bother me in the least. Of course, I had very little stimulation out there, and very little attachment. Attachment is what creates the fatigue. Now I sleep maybe 5½ to 6 hours, and then I can't sleep anymore. I get tired sometimes, but I watch why I'm getting tired and what the tiredness brings up in me.

RESOURCES

Books

Dass, R., and M. Bush. *Compassion in Action.* New York: Harmony/Crown, 1992.

_____. *Grist for the Mill.* Santa Cruz, CA: Unity Press, 1977.

_____. *Journey of Awakening.* New York: Bantam Books, 1978.

Organizations

Seva Foundation, 8 North San Pedro Road, San Rafael, CA 94903.

KARMA YOGA AND INNER PEACE
BY PEACE PILGRIM

When I started out, my hair had started to turn to silver. My friends thought I would surely kill myself, walking all over. But that didn't bother me. I just went ahead and did what I had to do. They didn't know that with inner peace I felt plugged into the source of universal energy, which never runs out. There was much pressure to compromise my beliefs, but I would not be dissuaded. Lovingly, I informed my well-meaning friends of the existence of two widely divergent paths in life and of the free will within all to make their choice.

There is a well-worn road which is pleasing to the senses and gratifies worldly desires, but leads to nowhere. And there is the less traveled path, which requires purifications and relinquishments, but results in untold spiritual blessings.

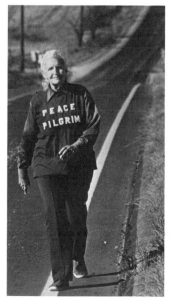

PEACE PILGRIM

. . .

It does not matter what name you attach to it, but your consciousness must ascend to the point through which you view the universe with your God-centered nature. The feeling accompanying this experience is that of complete oneness with the Universal Whole. One merges into a euphoria of absolute unity with all life: with humanity, with all the creatures of the earth, the trees and plants, the air, the water, and even earth itself. This God-centered nature is constantly awaiting to

217

govern your life gloriously. You have the free will to either allow it to govern your life, or not to allow it to affect you. This choice is always yours!

■ ■ ■

The path of the seeker is full of pitfalls and temptations, and the seeker must walk it alone with God. I would recommend that you keep your feet on the ground and your thoughts at lofty heights, so that you may attract only good. Concentrate on giving so that you may open yourself to receiving; concentrate on living according to the light you have so that you may open yourself to more light; get as much light as possible through the inner way. If such receiving seems difficult, look for some inspiration from a beautiful flower or a beautiful landscape, from some beautiful music or some beautiful words. However, that which is contacted from without must be confirmed within before it is yours.

■ ■ ■

I consider myself a server working on the *cause* of difficulties: *our immaturity.* And yet only a small minority are willing to work with cause. For every person working on cause there are thousands working on symptoms. I bless those who are working on the outer level to remove symptoms, but primarily I continue to work on the inner level to remove cause.

It is because most people have not found their purpose and function that they experience painful disharmony within, and thus the body of humanity is headed for chaos. Most of us fall short much more by omission than by commission: *"While the world perishes we go our way: purposeless, passionless, day after day."*

■ ■ ■

In my work I have chosen the positive approach. I never think of myself as protesting against something, but rather as *witnessing for* harmonious living. Those who witness *for*, present solutions. Those who witness *against*, usually do not—they dwell on what is wrong, resorting to judgment and criticism and sometimes even name-calling. Naturally, the negative approach has a detrimental effect on the person who uses it, while the positive approach has a good effect. When an evil is attacked, the evil mobilizes, although it may have been weak and unor-

Altruism is one of the glories of our human culture, and it must be learned just as we learn a language.

SIR JOHN ECCLES

True love is indivisible, it is always a transcendent. Because it "seeketh not itself to please," it alone justifies every delight. Yet the soul in us, because it has ever perfect Joy, never needs to seek for it, can only share and give.

LEWIS THOMPSON

ganized before, and therefore the attack gives it vitality and strength. When there is no attack, but instead good influences are brought to bear upon the situation, not only does the evil tend to fade away, but the evildoer tends to be transformed. The positive approach inspires; the negative approach makes angry. When you make people angry, they act in accordance with their baser instincts, often violently and irrationally. When you inspire people, they act in accordance with their higher instincts, sensibly and rationally. Also, anger is transient, whereas inspiration sometimes has a life-long effect.

■ ■ ■

There is a criterion by which you can judge whether the thoughts you are thinking and the things you are doing are right for you. The criterion is: *Have they brought you inner peace?* If they have not, there is something wrong with them—so keep seeking! If what you do has brought you inner peace, stay with what you believe is right.

■ ■ ■

When you find peace within yourself, you become the kind of person who can live at peace with others. Inner peace is not found by staying on the surface of life, or by attempting to escape from life through any means. Inner peace is found by facing life squarely, solving its problems, and delving as far beneath its surface as possible to discover its verities and realities. Inner peace comes through strict adherence to the already quite well known laws of human conduct, such as the law that the means shape the end: that only a good means can ever attain a good end. Inner peace comes through relinquishment of self-will, attachments, and negative thoughts and feelings. Inner peace comes through working for the good of all. We are all cells in the body of humanity— all of us, all over the world. Each one has a contribution to make, and will know from within what this contribution is, but no one can find inner peace except by working, not in a self-centered way, but for the whole human family.

Act in such a way that the totality of your will can always simultaneously serve as the foundation for law-making in general.

IMMANUEL KANT

The real mystic who has spiritual realizations or superconscious experiences becomes extremely interested in his fellow beings as he finds the expression of God in them. A mystic feels the presence of God everywhere and so he takes a loving interest not only in human beings but also in other beings.

SWAMI AKHILANANDA

WORK AND THE COSMIC BANK ACCOUNT
BY OMRAAM MIKHAEL AIVANHOV

Nothing can ever be gained without the sacrifice of something else. As the French have it: 'You can't make an omelette without breaking any eggs!' But I say, 'Yes, you can. It is possible to make an omelette without breaking any eggs. I know the secret!' . . . All you have to do is put all your capital in a bank on high and then, instead of growing weaker and exhausting yourself, the more you work the stronger and more powerful you become because, with every effort you make, something comes flowing into you to make up for what you have spent. But this will only happen, of course, if you place all your 'money,' all your 'capital' in a heavenly bank!

This is why it is so important that you should know whom you are working for and the goal you are aiming at, for it is this that determines the direction your energies will take. If, for instance, you are working for your father, you will not lose, you will gain. What counts most, therefore, is to know for what purpose you are spending your energies and in what direction you are working, for your future hangs on this: you are working either to impoverish or to enrich yourself.

Most people work unwittingly for an enemy concealed within who is robbing and despoiling them. A truly spiritual man is more intelligent; he works and spends his energies for someone who is really himself, and in this way it is he who gains. This is the intelligent thing to do: to become richer, not poorer. And it is not from selfishness or for the sake of his personality; on the contrary. Let's say, for instance, that you decide to work, not for yourself but for the collectivity. Well, since you are a member, an integral part of the collectivity, everything that improves and embellishes the collectivity will benefit each individual member of it, and this includes you. . . .

When I speak of "the collectivity" I am not speaking only of humanity, but of the whole universe, of all creatures in the universe and even of God Himself. This universal collectivity, this Immensity for which you are working, is like a bank, and all the work you do for it will come back to you, one day, increased many times over. For the universe does a very prosperous business; it is continually acquiring new constellations, new nebulae, new galaxies, and all this wealth will be yours. . . .

When you put some money into a bank, you don't receive the interest on it the very next day. You have to wait; and the longer you wait the more interest you get. And the same law applies in the spiritual domain. You may have been working with great love, patience, and faith, and, to begin with, you see no results. But don't be discouraged; if you give way to discouragement, it shows that you have not properly understood the laws that prevail on earth. Yes, indeed! You have to know the rules under which banking and administrations function. If you knew them you would realize that one always has to wait. In the long run, riches will

It is not necessary to go on a pilgrimage to find a sacred place, for one can create a sacred place wherever one is, the sacred space within. This involves clearing away the overwhelming trash and debris of self-imposed concerns, petty resentments and angers, the need to prove oneself right, mean competitiveness, litttle lies, taking advantage of people who are weaker and more defenseless, piling up money for its own sake, and all the other aids devised to puff up the ego.

JUNE SINGER

rain down on you from all sides; the whole universe will fling fabulous wealth at you. In fact, even if you wanted to avoid your reward, it would be impossible: you will have brought it all on yourself. It is a question of justice.

Note

[1]Swami Vivekananda, *Karma-Yoga and Bhakti-Yoga* (New York: Ramakrishna-Vivekananda Center, 1982), p. 37.

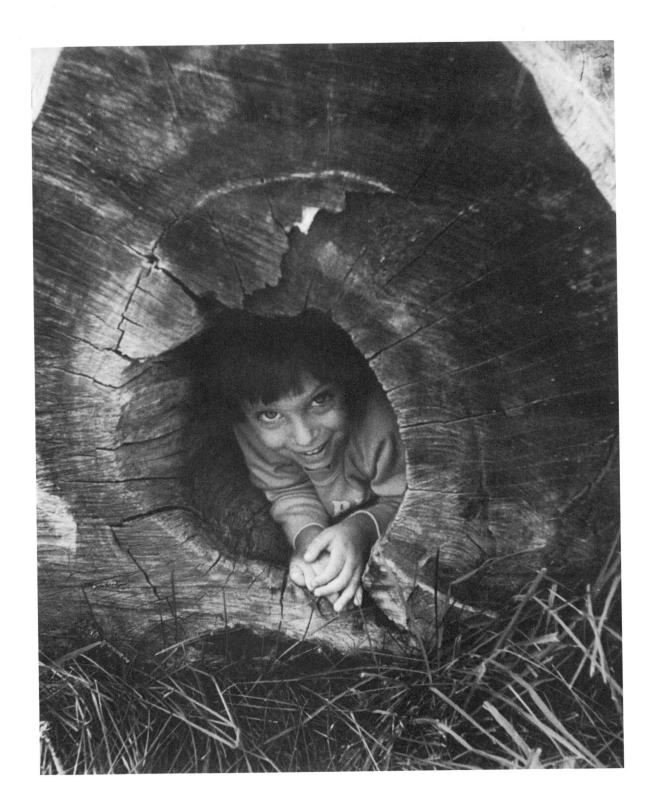

ELEVEN

Healing the Earth

During the past several decades it has become increasingly clear that we cannot truly heal ourselves so long as we have to live in an unhealthy environment. More and more, conscious people realize that the rapid industrialization and rising consumer expectations over the past 200 years have caused great damage to our planetary home, and that this blue world of ours is in need of deep healing. This ecological concern is now beginning to merge with the growing interest in personal growth and health. A new type of yoga is emerging: *eco-yoga*, which applies the universal moral and spiritual principles of the ancient yoga tradition to our modern situation. It seeks to reconnect us with the Earth and teaches us that we must find the sacred everywhere, not merely within ourselves.

We are pilgrims on this Earth, glimpsing the oneness of the sacred whole, knowing Gaia, knowing grace.

CHARLENE SPRETNAK

THE PRACTICE OF ECO-YOGA
BY GEORG FEUERSTEIN, PH.D.

All life is interconnected and ultimately interdependent. This living nexus is the subject-matter of ecology. Very simply, ecology is the study of the vital relationships between plants and animals (or humans) and the environment in which they live. Often the word is used to refer to the living being/environment connection itself.

Our planet has been likened to a gigantic spaceship whose resources are limited. While it is true that the Earth's resources are by no means inexhaustible, a far more important fact is that our home planet is

This whole cosmos is not just running on and running down for no meaning.

SIR JOHN ECCLES

vastly more complex than any technological device could ever be. It is, as biologist James Lovelock reminded our generation, a living organism, which he called Gaia. As a living organism, the Earth is a finely balanced system of forces.

Over the past several decades, this equilibrium has been seriously disturbed by unecological patterns of life characteristic mainly of the "civilized" countries of the world, leading to what is called the "ecological crisis." Many factors are involved in this very serious crisis, notably overpopulation, disadvantageous population distribution (e.g., huge metropolitan areas), overconsumption, wasteful patterns of consumption, inappropriate use of technology, and not least egocentric, short-sighted ways of thought.

What does all this have to do with yoga? Everything. Yoga is intrinsically ecological. All yoga is what I call "ego-yoga"—a term also used independently by philosopher Henryk Skolimowski. As the *Bhagavad Gita* (II.48), the oldest yoga scripture, puts it, yoga is balance. We need not understand this notion in purely psychological terms. Besides, when we are inwardly balanced, we are also balanced in relationship to our environment. This is borne out by the comprehensive and rigorous ethical code of yoga, which covers the whole range of the yoga practitioner's relationship to the environment and other living beings.

This code is expressed in the five rules of moral restraint. Thus, nonharming (ahimsa) consists in reverence for all forms of life. This implies, for instance, that we should choose a lifestyle that will not rob other creatures of their ecological niches. In fact, if we take this rule seriously, we must adopt a vegetarian diet. Failing this, we should ensure that our consumption of animal products (meat, eggs, and dairy products) at least does not in any way support the widespread cruel practice of factory-farming of animals.

The yogic rule of nonstealing (asteya) implies, for example, that we should not take more than we need for the upkeep of our body-mind. Few of us are willing to live in the Spartan fashion to which yogis are accustomed, but there are many things we can do to adapt to this moral obligation. Thus, we can avoid what has been called "conspicuous consumption," including the needless wasting of food. Instead, we could learn to simplify our life and also to use our surplus (which is often simply destined to become clutter and garbage) to improve the living conditions of our less fortunate fellow humans.

Similarly, the moral rule of greedlessness (aparigraha) is understood as a comprehensive demand to relate to life in a balanced, non-grasping manner, which respects the right of others to share the limited resources of our planet. Conscious living is a balance between giving and taking.

So, for instance, when we have to cut down a tree on our property, we should plant at least one new tree. Ego-yogic thinking demands that we help replenish our planet's resources.

The yogic call for purity (shauca), which is a part of the rules of self-discipline, can also be understood in a wide ecological sense. We should do our utmost to eliminate pollution in our own life and to support those efforts that seek to clean up our environment at large. Apart from any ethical consideration, pollution has become a major health hazard.

"Eco-yoga" refers to the now necessary convergence between traditional yogic spirituality and social activism focusing on ecological concerns. As we approach the end of the second millennium, we will face an increasing environmental crisis that will deeply affect all our lives. Thus, we cannot afford any longer to exclusively pursue quietistic goals. We must also take responsibility for the environment in which we live, and that means to recover our sense of the sacredness of this planet and to actively participate in its ecological recovery.

Metaphysically speaking, the challenge confronting us is to learn to respect both transcendence and immanence. To put it concretely, we cannot hope to find ourselves, never mind the Divine, as long as we obstruct our view by piling up mountains of garbage or by darkening the air with toxic pollutants. Instead, we must learn to cooperate with nature, which is the very basis for any spiritual effort we wish to make. We must be willing to be loyal not only to our chosen spiritual path but also to our habitat.

The tradition of Tantrism has hailed the body as a most valuable instrument for realizing the Divine, or Reality. We must similarly recognize the immense value of our planet. The Earth is our body, and it is the only one we have. If we destroy it, we destroy ourselves. If we honor it, we will be rewarded with plenty and well-being.

Here are some guidelines for cultivating the eco-yogic process:

1. Make a serious attempt at understanding our present age and the historical forces shaping it. Since we live in a complex pluralistic civilization, our lives are inevitably subject to all kinds of sociocultural currents,

According to integral yoga, Nature is no enemy of the spirit. On the contrary, she conceals the spirit in her bosom. As we cooperate with Nature, she affords us an ever-deepening insight into the glory of the spirit.

HARIDAS CHAUDHURI

which we need to understand in order to cultivate our own authenticity. In particular, we need to clearly comprehend the magnitude of the ecological crisis humanity is facing today. For a deeper understanding of the evolutionary potential of our time, I can heartily recommend *The Ever-Present Origin* by the Swiss cultural philosopher Jean Gebser; *The Aquarian Conspiracy* by Marilyn Ferguson; *Where the Wasteland Ends* by Theodore Roszak; and *The Passion of the Western Mind* by Richard Tarnas.

2. Become fully aware of, and informed about, the problem. Study books like Paul and Anne Ehrlich's *The Population Bomb* (1968) and *The Population Explosion* (1990); Barbara Ward's *The Home of Man* (1976); Thomas Berry's *The Dream of the Earth* (1988); Duane Elgin's *Voluntary Simplicity* (1981); Mihajlo Mesarovic's and Eduard Pestel's Club-of-Rome report *Mankind at the Turning Point* (1974); Jonathon Porritt's *Seeing Green* (1984); Lester Brown's ongoing *State of the World* reports; the Sierra Club's *Ecotactics* (1970), edited by John G. Mitchell and Constance L. Stallings; and *The Greenhouse Trap* (1990), edited by Francesca Lyman et al. All these publications, and many other good books, contain a wealth of valuable information that has immediate relevance. But there are a few books that can be particularly recommended as practical manuals: *The Global Ecology Handbook: What You Can Do About the Environmental Crisis* (1990), edited by Walter H. Corson; *50 Simple Things You Can Do to Save the Earth* (1989), *50 Simple Things Kids Can Do to Save the Earth* (1990); *The Recycler's Handbook* (1990) by the EarthWorks Group, in Berkeley, California; and *The Simple Act of Planting a Tree* (1990) by Treepeople, with Andy and Katie Lipkis.

You don't have to become an expert, but you ought to know what is happening around you that affects you and the life of your children.

3. Live a simpler, ecologically sensitive life. Take stock of your consumption patterns and decide how you can help reduce energy consumption and pollution in your own immediate environment. For instance, ask yourself: Do I need to have so many lights on? Do I really need to run the air conditioner or heater, or could I insulate my house better and thus cut down energy wastage? Do I need to use the car quite so often, or could I plan my trips more wisely and perhaps use car pools? Do I need to flush the toilet with every use, or have fifteen-minute showers every day? Why couldn't I recycle cans and bottles? Can I really not afford to buy healthier organic food? Am I simply too lethargic to use vegetable waste to make a compost pile in the garden? And so on. Big change begins by doing the "little" things—now.

4. Join forces with a local ecology group and become politically active. Yoga is not merely inwardness. Nor are yoga practice and political commitment incompatible. All too often yoga practitioners are concerned with their own salvation, ignoring the larger context in which they live. In the final analysis, this is not only selfish and contrary to the spirit of yoga but also counterproductive. For, the environment impinges on us. For example, how can you hope to cultivate breath control in a polluted neighborhood? Or how can you hope to maintain a healthy body-mind when the soil on which your food grows is poisoned by chemicals? Or how can you hope to achieve the necessary inner stillness for meditation and prayer to transform your psyche when your eardrums vibrate from the constant cacophony on the streets and in the sky?

At the very least, support activist groups like Greenpeace, Friends of the Earth, Sierra Club, Nature Conservancy, and the Elmwood Institute.

For the individual, with no tribe and an illusory nation, what allegiance is there, except to a global community? This is not a coincidence, but a natural pattern of evolution, involving individuation, integration, and unification—from individuated ego to collective "super" ego to the unified ego of earthmind.

MICHAEL W. FOX

5. Cultivate self-understanding by scrutinizing the motives behind your spiritual odyssey, and be willing to recognize and work with neurotic tendencies masquerading as spiritual ideals. This is a form of jnana yoga. Don't necessarily trust your own insights but consult benevolent others who may serve you as a more accurate mirror of your own character. Inadequate self-understanding frequently leads to wrong action.

6. Study the spiritual traditions of the world to deepen your understanding of your preferred path. This will help you appreciate the complementarity of the Earth's religious and spiritual traditions. It will also reduce the tendency toward parochialism, cultism, spiritual elitism, and other forms of exclusivism. Such study can help you cultivate the admirable and indeed essential virtues of compassion and tolerance, which facilitate cooperation and ecological living.

7. Stay in touch with your natural environment. Living in cities seduces people into having a merely abstract relationship to the Earth. It is important to touch the soil, tend flowers or trees, taste clean spring water, see the exuberance of wildlife, and so on. Inwardness without such grounding is often little more than neurotic escape. Wholeness requires the transformative touch of the Earth as well as the blessing from the "heaven within."

8. Daily remind yourself that life is a precious gift, which must not be squandered. If your heart is open, gratitude and praise will flow easily from your lips. Our Western upbringing, generally speaking, does not make us predisposed to express our gratitude (or our other emotions), and it teaches us to be critical rather than full of praise. There is, of course, no need to withhold criticism where it is due, but it is often received more readily when it is tempered with compassion and praise (which can be viewed as an active form of compassion).

Living in our postmodern world has wounded us all in one way or another, and there is much need for healing. Praise and the expression of gratitude are, in my experience, an excellent means of soothing our pain and restoring hope. When we experience life as a spiritual opportunity for which we are grateful, the world ceases to be our enemy. We will still share in the harvest of our collective karma and feel sorrow at the exploitation of the Earth, but we will also begin to feel a deeper affinity for everyone and everything, which is healing in itself. We become true ecological citizens of the world, true eco-yogis.

DEEP ECOLOGY
BY TANYA KUCAK

Water that poisons, air that chokes, noise that deadens sensibilities— the signs of environmental degradation and imminent disaster are everywhere. Yet glimmers of hope are still to be found. Rain after a long drought brings forth sprigs of green. The fertile soil that follows a fire fosters bright-colored blossoms. And a radical change in our attitudes toward and relationship with nature may yet re-create clean water, fragrant air, and silences punctuated by birdsong. The attitudes needed for this radical change are reflected in the philosophy of deep ecology.

Indeed, deep ecology informs us that we are a part of the natural world in the deepest and most intimate sense, each of us a cell in the

In relation to the earth, we have been autistic for centuries. Only now have we begun to listen with some attention and with a willingness to respond to the earth's demands that we cease our industrial assault, that we abandon our inner rage against the conditions of our earthly existence, that we renew our human participation in the grand liturgy of the universe.

THOMAS BERRY

organism called nature. It follows that we must apply the Golden Rule in our dealings with nature, and do unto Nature as we would have nature do unto us.

That this is a radical shift is obvious when we consider the acres of farmland paved over for highways, the fruit orchards converted to parking lots, shopping centers, and factories, and the clean, still air despoiled by our modes of transportation.

The Problem

Our environmental problems stem largely from our underlying cultural assumptions about nature. Philosophically, these assumptions, as articulated by Warwick Fox in *The Ecologist* (Sept./Oct. 1984), fall into three categories.

Spirituality now flowers from the very roots and seeds of this planet. It does not have to be brought anymore by emissaries from outer space.

ROBERT MULLER

1. Man is the measure of all things. (Historically, this has meant only men, not women—perhaps in part because women could not ignore the cycles of nature so easily.) The boundaries between man and nature are sharp and distinct. Moreover, not only is the nonhuman world subservient to the human world, but its value is gauged in terms of its usefulness to men.

2. As in the classical Greek and Cartesian views of the universe, the world is atomistic, divisible, nonrelativistic, and comprehensible only by a reductionistic approach. Mechanical metaphors describe the world. Things in nature are separate and distinct from each other as well as from us. Nature is inert: trees are static, rocks are dead.

3. Economic growth is unquestioned. Wilderness areas are managed, mined, and logged. Nature becomes an economic resource, susceptible to management. Growth and development are the primary considerations.

These attitudes help explain why most attempts to solve environmental problems have been largely ineffective. The underlying cultural assumptions predispose us to shallow, short-term solutions that are overwhelmingly anthropocentric, treat environmental problems as if they were disconnected, and favor economics over nature.

What Is Deep Ecology?

According to Norwegian philosopher Arne Naess, who coined the term, "the essence of deep ecology [as distinguished from shallow ecology, which is the usual, short-term view of nature] is to ask deeper questions. The adjective 'deep' stresses that we ask why and how, where others do not." Furthermore, "we ask which society, which education, which form of religion, is beneficial for all life on the planet as a whole, and then we ask further what we need to do . . . to make the necessary changes."[1]

Warwick Fox has articulated some of the social, political, and economic concepts associated with deep ecology: a just and sustainable society; frugality; dwelling in place or developing a sense of place; cultural and biological diversity; local autonomy and decentralization; renewable energy; and appropriate technology. To live by these principles, we would have to assume a smaller-scale, slower-paced lifestyle attuned to the rhythms of nature, not to those of commerce or clockwork.

Parallel to the three underlying assumptions of classical Western views toward nature are three underlying assumptions of deep ecology.

1. Human beings are just one species among others in the community of nature, and they are not separate from their environment. All living beings are intrinsically equal.

2. Everything is connected, and the interrelationships are constantly changing. The world is dynamic, fluid, and interdependent. As in the "new" physics, observers affect what they observe. The natural world is pantheistic, and the metaphors are biological, rather than mechanistic.

3. Instead of economic growth, this view assumes ecological sustainability and requires a long-term view, as well as an understanding of such ecological concepts as diversity and symbiosis. Many deep ecologists favor vast *unmanaged* wilderness rather than developed wilderness areas. Not only is untamed wilderness valuable in itself, they maintain—some species can flourish only when undisturbed—but it is valuable for spiritual reasons as well. As Thoreau put it, in his 1862 essay "Walking," "In wildness is the preservation of the world."

John Seed, founder of the Rainforest Information Centre, makes explicit his spiritual connection with nature when he states in his essay "Think Like a Mountain": "I am that part of the rainforest recently emerged into thinking." Seed also points out the continuum between living and lifeless when he says poetically: "We are the rocks dancing."

This sort of pantheistic, intimate embrace of nature harkens back to so-called primitive societies, where nature did have faces, animals were totems, and rocks had character.

Gary Snyder, in *The Old Ways*, advises us to cultivate patience and attention so that we can relearn some of the wisdom our ancestors practiced in their daily lives. Part of that wisdom is to know the place you inhabit, to develop "a much deeper knowledge and self-sufficiency related to the plants, animals, weather patterns, the lore of the place . . . first and foremost, I think, to know plants." Snyder wants us to regain "the capacity to hear the song of Gaia *at that spot*."

Cultivating a deep ecological consciousness, then, is a first step toward healing our relationship with nature and recovering the wisdom we need to live in harmony with nature.

Nature is made to conspire with spirit to emancipate us.

RALPH WALDO EMERSON

RESOURCES

Books and Articles

Anderson, L., ed. *Sisters of the Earth*. New York: Vintage Books, 1991.

Berry, T. *The Dream of the Earth*. San Francisco: Sierra Club Books, 1988.

Corson, W. H. *The Global Ecology Handbook: What You Can Do About the Environmental Crisis*. Boston, MA: Beacon Press, 1990.

Devall, B., and G. Sessions. *Deep Ecology: Living as If Nature Mattered*. Salt Lake City, UT: Peregrine Smith Books, 1985.

Fox, M. W. *Toward a Transpersonal Ecology: Developing New Foundations for Environmentalism*. Boston, MA: Shambhala, 1990.

Leon, G., D. Hinrichsen, and A. Markham. *Atlas of the Environment*. New York: Prentice Hall, 1990.

Naess, A. *Ecology, Community, and Lifestyle: Outline of an Ecosophy*. New York: Cambridge University Press, 1989.

Seed, J., J. Macy, P. Fleming, and A. Naess. *Thinking Like a Mountain: Toward a Council of All Beings.* Philadelphia, PA: New Society Publishers, 1988.

Skolimowski, H. *Eco-Philosophy: Designing New Tactics for Living.* London and Salem, NH: Marion Boyars, 1981.

Snyder, G. *The Old Ways.* San Francisco: City Lights Books, 1977.

Thoreau, H. D. *The Portable Thoreau.* New York: Viking, 1947.

Tobias, M., ed. *Deep Ecology.* San Marcos, CA: Avant Books, 1985.

Periodicals

The following two publications are most likely to carry articles on deep ecology:

The Ecologist magazine, published bimonthly in England; U.S. distributor: MIT Press, 55 Hayward Street, Cambridge, MA 02142-1399.

Resurgence magazine, published bimonthly in England; U.S. distributor: Rodale Press, 33E Minor Street, Emmaus, PA 18098-0099.

World Watch. Published bimonthly by the Worldwatch Institute, 1776, Massachusetts Avenue NW, Washington, DC 20036.

Also useful are:

Earth Ethics newsletter. Published quarterly by the Center for Respect of Life and Environment, 2100 L Street NW, Washington, DC 20037.

EarthSave newsletter. Published quarterly and available to members of EarthSave, 706 Frederick Street, Santa Cruz, CA 95062.

Garbage: The Practical Journal for the Environment, published bimonthly by Old House Journal Corporation, 2 Main Street, Gloucester, MA 01930.

Organizations

Rainforest Information Centre, c/o Ian Peter, P.O. Box 368, Lismore, NSW 2480, Australia.

Rocky Mountain Institute, 1739 Snowmass Creek Road, Snowmass, CO 81654. Tel. (303) 927-3128.

PRAYER FOR THE GREAT FAMILY
BY GARY SNYDER

Gratitude to Mother Earth, sailing through night and day—
and to her soil: rich, rare, and sweet
in our minds so be it.

Gratitude to Plants, the sun-facing, light-changing leaf
and fine root-hairs; standing still through wind
and rain; their dance is in the flowing spiral grain
in our minds so be it.

Gratitude to Air, bearing the soaring Swift and the silent
Owl at dawn. Breath of our song
clear spirit breeze
in our minds so be it.

Gratitude to Wild Beings, our brothers, teaching secrets,
freedoms, and ways; who share with us their milk;
self-complete, brave, and aware
in our minds so be it.

Gratitude to Water. clouds, lakes, rivers, glaciers;
holding or releasing; streaming through all
our bodies salty seas
in our minds so be it.

Gratitude to the Sun: blinding pulsing light through
trunks of trees, through mists, warming caves where
bears and snakes sleep—he who wakes us—
in our minds so be it.

Gratitude to the Great Sky
who holds billions of stars—and goes yet beyond that—
beyond all powers, and thoughts
and yet is within us—
Grandfather Space.
The Mind is his Wife.

so be it.

—After a Mohawk prayer

*Awe at the intricate wonders of
creation and celebration of the
cosmic unfolding are the roots
of worship.*

CHARLENE SPRETNAK

THINK LIKE A MOUNTAIN
BY JOHN SEED

Anthropocentrism, or human chauvinism—the idea that human beings are the crown of creation, the source of all value, the measure of all things—is deeply embedded in our culture and consciousness.

> And the fear of you and the dread of you shall be upon every beast of the earth, and upon every fowl of the air, and upon all that moveth on the earth, and upon all the fishes of the sea; into your hands they are delivered. (Genesis 9:2)

When humans finally start to see through their layers of anthropocentric self-cherishing, a most profound change in consciousness begins to take place. The result has sometimes been referred to as "deep ecology," a term coined by Norwegian philosopher and eco-activist Arne Naess.

When we embrace this view, alienation subsides. The human is no longer an outsider, apart. Humanness is then recognized as being merely the most recent stage of our existence, and as we stop identifying exclusively with this chapter in our evolution, we begin to get in touch with ourselves as mammals, as vertebrates, as a species only recently emerged from the rainforest. As the fog of amnesia disperses, there is a transformation in our relationship to other species, and in our commitment to taking care of them.

What is described here should not be seen as merely intellectual. The intellect is one entry point to the process outlined, and the easiest one to communicate. For some people, however, this change of perspective follows from actions on behalf of Mother Earth.

"I am protecting the rainforest" develops into "I am part of the rainforest protecting myself. I am that part of the rainforest recently emerged into thinking." This change in perspective is spiritual more than intellectual.

With this new perspective on creation, we begin to recall our true nature. As the memory improves, as the implications of evolution and ecology are internalized and replace the outmoded anthropocentric structures in the mind, we begin to identify with all life. Then follows the realization that the distinction between "life" and "lifeless" is a human construct. Every atom in the human body existed before organic life emerged 4,000 million years ago. One may even remember one's previous existence as minerals, as lava, as rocks.

As long as our thinking is exclusively self-centered the world will remain fragmented.

JEAN GEBSER

234

Rocks contain the potential to weave themselves into such stuff as this. We are the rocks dancing. Why do we look down on them with such a condescending air? It is they that are the immortal part of us.

If we embark upon such an inner voyage, we may find, upon returning to consensus reality, that our actions on behalf of the environment are purified and strengthened by the experience.

We have found here a level of our being that moths, rust, nuclear holocaust, or destruction of the genepools cannot corrupt. Our commitment to save the world is not decreased by this new perspective, although the fear and anxiety that were part of our motivation start to dissipate and are replaced by a certain disinterestedness. We act not only because life is the only game in town, but also because actions from a disinterested, less attached consciousness are more effective. This disinterestedness or non-attachment has much in common with meditation. And since most activists don't have much time for meditation, this perspective becomes an effective substitute. In fact, more and more teachers of meditation are embracing "deep ecology."

According to Naess, "the essence of deep ecology is to ask deeper questions. . . We ask which society, which education, which form of religion, is beneficial for all life on the planet as a whole."

Of all the species that have ever existed, it is estimated that less than one in a hundred exist today. The rest became extinct because as environment changes, any species that is unable to adapt, to change, to evolve, is extinguished. All evolution takes place in this fashion. In this way our ancestor, an oxygen-starved fish, commenced to colonize the land. Threat of extinction is the potter's hand that molds all life forms.

The human species is one of millions threatened by imminent extinction through nuclear war and other environmental changes. And while it is true that the "human nature" revealed by 12,000 years of written history does not offer much hope that we can change our warlike, greedy, ignorant ways, the vastly longer fossil history assures us that we *can*. We *are* that fish, and the myriad other death-defying feats of flexibility that a study of evolution reveals to us. In spite of our recent "humanity," a certain confidence is warranted.

From this point of view, the threat of extinction appears as the invitation to change, to evolve. After a brief respite from the potter's hand, here we are back on the wheel again. The change that is required of us this time is not some new resistance to radiation, but a change in consciousness. Deep ecology is the search for that consciousness.

Surely, consciousness emerged and evolved according to the same

The earth can no longer be owned; it must be shared.

MURRAY BOOKCHIN

235

laws as everything else—molded by environmental pressures. In the recent past, when faced with intolerable environmental pressures, the mind of our ancestors must time and again have been forced to transcend itself.

To survive our current environmental crisis, we must consciously remember our evolutionary and ecological inheritance. We must learn, according to Arne Naess, to think like a mountain. If we are to be open to evolving a new consciousness, we must fully face up to our impending extinction (the ultimate environmental pressure). . . . This means acknowledging the part of us that shies away from the truth and hides in intoxication or busyness from the despair of the human species, whose 4,000-million-year race is run, whose organic life is a mere hair's breadth from finished.

A biocentric perspective, the realization that rocks *will* dance, and that roots go deeper than 4,000 million years, may give us the courage to face despair and break through to a more viable consciousness, one that is sustainable and in harmony with life again.

What yearns to be big in us, to be vast beyond reckoning, is the adventure of self-discovery. The larger that grows, the more lightly human society will rest upon the earth.

THEODORE ROSZAK

GUARDIANS OF GAIA
BY JOANNA MACY

For thou shalt be in league with the stones of the field, and the beasts of the field shall be at peace with thee.

JOB 5:23

This verse from the Bible delighted me as a child and stayed with me as I grew up. It promised a way I wanted to live—in complicity with creation. It still comes to mind when I hear about people taking action on behalf of other species. When our brothers and sisters of Greenpeace or Earth First! put their lives on the line to save the whales or the old-growth forests, I think, "Ah, they're in league."

To be "in league" in that way seems wonderful to me. There is a comfortable, cosmic collegiality to it—like coming home to conspire once more with our beloved and age-old companions, with the stones and the beasts of the field, and the sun that rises and the stars that wheel in the sky.

Now the work of restoring our ravaged Earth offers us that—and with a new dimension. It puts us in league not only with the stones and the beasts, but also with the beings of the future. All that we do for the mending of our planet is for their sakes, too. Their chance to live in and love our world depends in large measure on us and our often uncertain efforts.

At gatherings and workshops that address the ecological or nuclear crisis, we often begin with an evocation of the "beings of the three times." We invited their presence at our deliberations. In evoking beings of the past and the present, we take time to speak their names, spontaneously and at random—names of ancestors and teachers who cherished this Earth, then names of those living now, with whom we work and share this time of danger. But after the third evocation, which calls on the beings of future time, there is silence: for we do not know their names. Yet that moment of silence is the most potent of all to me, for those unborn ones are so many, and so innocent, and so at our mercy. . . .

The imagined presence of these futures ones comes to me like grace, and works upon my life.

Note

[1] All quotes by Arne Naess are from "Simple in Means, Rich in Ends: A Conversation with Arne Naess," by Stephan Bodian (*Ten Directions*, Summer/Fall 1982).

PART FIVE

RITUAL AND BEYOND: TANTRA YOGA

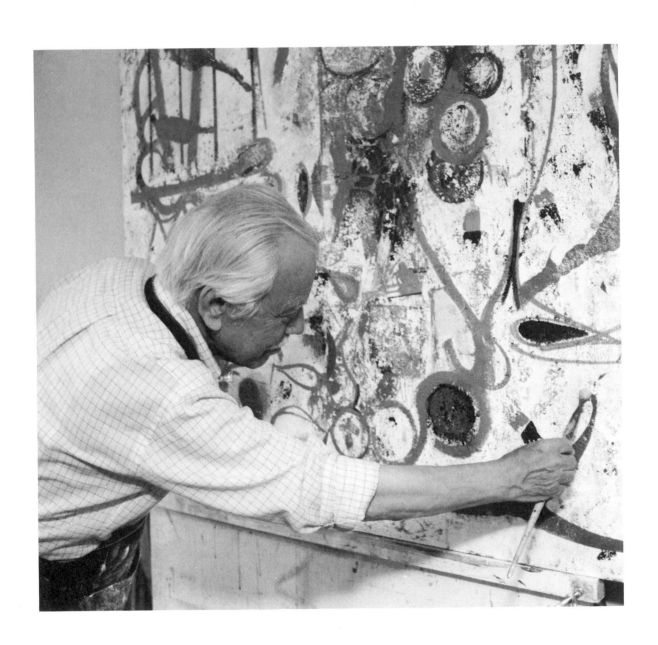

TWELVE

The Creative Spirit

Tantra yoga is the most misunderstood branch of the yoga tradition. It is widely confused with sexual rituals, performed to achieve altered states of mind. In fact, tantra yoga is the path of ritual as such, and sexual rituals form only a small part of this yogic orientation. Tantra yoga is about realizing that our personal creativity is rooted in, or derives from, cosmic creative potential itself. From the tantric perspective, creativity is a manifestation of the feminine principle of the universe, the Goddess, called *shakti*.

In this chapter, we will look at creativity and how it can be used to put us in touch with the sacred dimension of existence. Rituals are a significant aspect of creativity, and they are here presented as principal means of focusing attention on the spiritual process. You will learn how to incorporate useful rituals into your daily life, so you can punctuate your day with periodic reminders of the sacred presence that suffuses everything and everybody.

To me, "noncreative intelligence" is a flat-out contradiction in terms.

DOUGLAS R. HOFSTADTER

YOGA AS SACRED ART

There is a widespread belief that spiritual life and creativity are incompatible, that in order to grow as spiritual beings we must flee the world and deny our creative impulses. This notion is found in the tradition of radical world-denial and asceticism. While there are schools within the yoga tradition that subscribe to this notion, there are many more schools that avow a life-affirmative orientation.

241

For instance, in the great cultural movement of Tantrism we encounter the belief that the universe itself is a manifestation of the Divine, and that therefore the human being is an expression of the creative superabundance of the ultimate Reality. So, for the practitioners of Tantrism (or Tantra), the body is a temple of the Divine, and for this reason we must approach life and embodiment with reverence.

The world is, for them, the playground of the Goddess (Shakti). What appears to the ordinary person as inert matter is, upon awakening, a marvelously dynamic field of energy—the Goddess. Tantric yoga is always an attempt to enlist the help of that cosmic feminine principle and, ultimately, to unite with it in the state of ecstasy.

Tantrism emerged in India in the early post-Christian centuries, though its roots reach back into the remote past. The many teachers of this movement sought to bring about a positive reevaluation of existence. For them, the sacred was to be found everywhere—in everyone and in everything. Because of this orientation, they were able to freely utilize all aspects of human life in their quest for spiritual freedom and spontaneity.

The Tantric teachers were masters of ritual. They understood that the human mind could be disciplined and transcended through the repeated performance of symbolic actions. Ritual is action that is charged with symbolic significance and that connects the individual to the sacred reality. It is action that is performed by intensely remembering the superlative creativity of the Goddess, the divine energy weaving the universe. Ritual is always creative.

By contrast, routine action, which is of course also repetitive, lacks conscious symbolism and intention and is decidedly uncreative. Ritual dies when it becomes dull routine or enforced duty. For ritual to remain meaningful and constructive, we must engage it wholeheartedly. This means we must be present as and through the body, rather than dissociate from it. Ritual calls for the union of body, mind, and spirit.

All yoga practice has at its core the endeavor to move beyond the ego-personality, beyond mere routine existence. In this sense, the yogic discipline is inherently ritualistic and creative. Through it, we invite the Goddess, the creative spirit, into our lives. Genuine yoga always implicates our whole existence, affecting all aspects of our life. It is a way of living creatively in the sacred presence. Whatever our occupation or our task at hand, through yoga we can render all our actions and thoughts sacred. Indeed, this creative ritual of infusing the light of the spirit into our life is the quintessence of all spirituality.

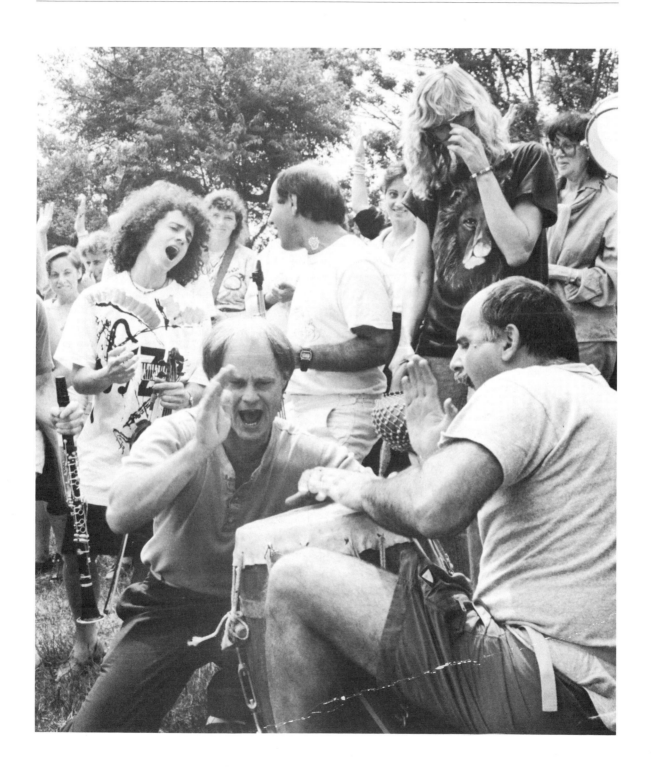

Practitioners of yoga are true artists. They are constantly creating a new and better destiny for themselves—a destiny that gradually liberates them from selfish interests and brings them closer and closer to the blissful center of the sacred reality.

REMEMBERING THE DEEPER MEANING OF CELEBRATION
BY CAROLYN R. SHAFFER

Together we chanted, holding hands and letting the drumbeat enter into our bodies on a cellular level, reminding us of the heartbeat of Mother Earth, beating, beating for life. We need to keep up the cermonies, sisters and brothers.

VICKI NOBLE

Today, our science-based culture has effectively discarded the sacred and collapsed consensual reality into a single, factual, measurable dimension. Without sacred time or space, we find ourselves looking out upon the vast, featureless expanse of the ordinary. No wonder we have trouble celebrating. Our culture doesn't tell us how to distinguish between mundane and festival time. All we know for sure is that occasionally we get time off work for a holiday. But what does a holiday, or "holy day," mean in a culture that doesn't recognize the sacred?

In earlier days in Europe—and among indigenous, agricultural cultures throughout the Northern Hemisphere today—many of the public, communal rites celebrated the changing of the seasons. Even the Christian rites borrowed heavily from the nature-based celebrations that preceded them. Participants viewed reality as cyclical or spiral. Celebrations marked the end of one natural cycle and the beginning of another, a moment when ordinary time stopped and the sacred or numinous broke through.

We industrialized North Americans know little of cycles. Our factories operate around the clock, and our supermarkets stay open 24 hours a day. What's more, our culture expects us to operate at peak performance at all times. We're not considered successful unless we're constantly growing, moving up, getting richer. In a linear, clock-driven culture such as this, how do we take time out to celebrate? And what does celebration mean when there is apparently no other reality to cross over to?

When properly performed, celebrations, like the moon or the cycle of the year, have phases. French folklorist Arnold van Gennep, in his seminal book *The Rites of Passage*, labeled the three major phases of ritual as *separation* or preliminal, *margin* or liminal, and *reaggregation* or postliminal. ("Liminal" comes from the Latin word *limen*, meaning "threshold.") In the first phase, participants prepare for entry into another reality; in the second, they enter this sacred time and space and are transformed or reborn by the act of crossing the threshold; and, in the third, they return changed to ordinary reality—and usually throw a party.

In our contemporary Euro-American culture, we tend to skip the first two phases and just throw the party. Nothing sacred or cyclical about it. Unfortunately, there's also nothing celebratory about it, since celebration is inextricably linked with the sacred.

The sacred, writes Mircea Eliade in his classic work *The Sacred and the Profane*, "is an absolute reality . . . which transcends this world but manifests itself in this world, thereby sanctifying it and making it real." Genuine celebration, according to Eliade, doesn't merely honor an event or accomplishment, but, like the Hopi new year ceremony known as Soyal, it re-creates the world.

Reducing a celebration to a party is like presenting the Oscar awards on television without bothering to make the movies. We celebrate but know not what we are honoring. The party becomes simply a momentary diversion with no connection to past or future, much less to the mythic dimension of life.

If man is to survive, I believe he must undergo the agony of the Dromenon—the dancing, stretching, dying and re-membering of himself beyond his conditioned social and cultural limitations.

JEAN HOUSTON

RITUAL IN DAILY LIFE
BY RENEE BECK

For those of us seeking to create balance within ourselves and on our planet, ritual can be an effective tool. Ritual has been used for thousands of years to honor important events in our lives: to give passion and boldness to beginnings; to sanctify and strengthen mergings; to deepen our participation in the cyclical turnings in our lives and in our world; to embrace and nourish us in endings; and to heal us when we feel pain or isolation.

Ritual, the use of symbols and meaningful actions fired by intention toward a specific purpose, can afford a means of entry into sacred time and space, an access to meaning in life and the tattoo of daily routine. We so easily become polarized in only one aspect of who we are—be it thought, feeling, or action—that we lose track of the bigger picture. Just as the practice of yoga strives for the balanced union of all aspects of the self, so too can ritual create this sense of wholeness by the use of symbols.

Symbols are the language of the unconscious, just as words are the language of the conscious mind. We all have symbols that are personally meaningful and images that arouse feeling on a collective cultural level (such as a national flag). Images from dreams and myths can affect

*We are all one in the spirit and
in the body. . . . The purpose
of ceremony is to bring an
awareness of such unity into
consciousness. It is a necessary
component of the human learning
process, yet now it must be
relearned.*

SEDONIA CAHILL AND
JOSHUA HALPERN

us on a deep level, one that feels larger than who we are, because they tap into the collective unconscious—that part of our being which is shared by all humans. The archetypes, or psychic structures derived from common human experience, are found in the collective unconscious, and their symbols are seen universally, although in different forms. For example, all cultures have symbols of birth and death, of good and evil, of the hero and his journey, of the savior, and of the mother and child. The collective unconscious, an enormous reservoir of knowledge and power, can be accessed by the intentional use of such symbols.

Of particular relevance and potency are those symbols that represent the elements we see in nature: earth, water, air, and fire. Our world is fueled by the sun (fire), whose heat is contained by the atmosphere (air). We are nourished by the depths and rhythms of the ocean and rain (water), which bring forth life from the ground on which we also move and build our lives (earth). The balanced interaction of these elements can be seen as nature (spirit). These elements also exist within ourselves, as energy (fire), mind (air), emotions (water), and body (earth), which, when balanced, facilitate the sense of wholeness, or the connectedness of the centerpoint of Self with all points of the circle of existence (spirit).

The practice of yoga itself reflects the four elements: will (fire) is needed to carry out the discipline, to energize a sometimes recalcitrant body (earth) to perform the postures and movements (water). The breath (air) is used to communicate the will to the body. If yoga is approached as a ritual, the intention (fire) is to balance body (earth), thoughts (air), and feelings (water) in union (spirit) with the inner self. The body, the asanas and mudras, and the breath are the primary symbols, but other symbols and symbolic acts are involved as well.

Thus, going to your place of practice or beginning a yoga session can be viewed as entering sacred time/space. Your mat or towel may be seen as an "altar cloth," further defining the space as sacred and the actions to be performed upon it as more than mundane. Reverential acts toward your teacher can be symbolic honorings of the balance and union you strive for within yourself. Overcoming mental, emotional, or physical blocks to accomplish a difficult yogic practice is indeed reflective of the hero's journey. Ending exercises and rolling up your practice mat represent closure and a return to normal existence (although, as with any effective ritual, the experience comes with you, enhancing your daily life). Even without making yoga a ritual, by being conscious of these symbols, both your practice and your sense of the sacred can deepen.

Bringing this symbol-sensitive consciousness into other areas of your life can also help you achieve harmony and union. Every act can be a sacred act, without the need for elaborate rituals requiring great planning, props, and presentation. Breakfast, for instance, can be a ritual, by consciously attending to it with the intention of creating balance within yourself for the day ahead. In firing up the kettle, you are seeking equilibrium between your passion (fire) and your emotions (water); the food you eat can symbolize strength and right action (earth) throughout the day; you can use your morning yawns to symbolize clearing your thoughts (air). The roundness of your plate or cup can represent the oneness of spirit from which you receive sustenance, as can interacting with your family around the breakfast table.

Rituals need not be fancy. Indeed, some of the simplest rituals can be very profound and effective: lighting a candle to represent spirit and acknowledging the four directions as aspects of the Self—east/air/mind; south/fire/energy; west/water/emotions; and north/earth/body.

We also can bring deeper meaning to the rituals we already practice, by going into them with intention. For example, a traditional birthday party can be enhanced by adding a few simple touches. Begin by asking the blessing of spirit (or God, Goddess, Love, the One, etc.) with the lighting of the candles (fire). Standing in a circle (spirit) around the celebrant and cake, people make toasts (air) to her, which she symbolically drinks (water). People sing "Happy Birthday," giving the celebrant their love (water) and energy (fire) that she may blow out (air) all the candles, so that her intentions for the year may manifest. She cuts and eats the birthday cake (earth) to ground these intentions, incorporating them into the life of her body. The participants can also use the celebration to reaffirm to themselves their own yearly intentions.

The art of ritual consists not so much in the showmanship and weightiness we often associate with many of our culture's formal rituals, but in intention and in the awareness and use of the symbols that are always within and around us. It is the nature of human beings to grow and to increase our relationships with ourselves, each other, our world, and the spirit. It is in this that the true substance of our lives is based; it is contact with this moving essence that makes the difference between merely existing and fully living, between wishing for change and being able to create true change within ourselves and our world. Ritual is one way to reconnect with this essence.

When there's no self-interest involved in what you do, then a lot of the chemicals in your system don't get engaged. When those chemicals aren't present, then your ego doesn't have its usual relationship to the activity. It's a wonderful opportunity to explore pure action—to be aware of it and to feel it.

SWAMI CHETANANANDA

RESOURCES

Books

Beck, R., and S. B. Metrick. *The Art of Ritual*. Berkeley, CA: Celestial Arts, 1990.

Cahill, S., and J. Halpern. *Ceremonial Circle: Practice, Ritual, and Renewal for Personal and Community Healing*. San Francisco: HarperSanFrancisco, 1992.

Starhawk. *The Spiral Dance: A Rebirth of the Ancient Religion of the Great Goddess*. San Francisco: Harper & Row, 1989.

van Gennep, A. *The Rites of Passage*. Chicago: University of Chicago Press, 1960.

The power to create and foster harmony is greater than the power to destroy and bring chaos.

ANDREW BARD
SCHMOOKLER

THE CREATIVE SPIRIT
BY ANNE CUSHMAN

When I was a child, I loved to tell myself stories. For hours I would lie entranced on my bedroom floor, clutching a handful of Popsicle sticks (the magic talismans that would start the torrent of tales) and recounting the adventures of imaginary characters who became my closest friends. Occasionally, as I grew older, I wrote the stories down, sometimes illustrating them with crayons or magic markers. I always threw them away when I was done. The stories themselves didn't matter—it was the act of creating them that was essential.

But then I got an education. I went to good schools and learned about art and literature, about symbols, metaphors, and style. I realized how trivial my creative efforts were, compared to the work of the great masters. Besides, writing critical essays and studying for exams left no time for playing with Popsicle sticks. Halfway through high school, I picked up a handful of Popsicle sticks and realized I no longer even knew how.

My experience is not unusual. For most of us, the extravagant creativity of childhood is soon crushed by the demands of parents, schools, and society. At an early age, we come to believe that artistic talent is a finite substance randomly doled out at birth to a blessed few. Certain rare individuals are inspired by the Muse, we are informed. The rest of us are fated to be nothing but *consumers* of art: decorating our houses with other people's paintings, playing other people's songs on our stereos, munching stale popcorn as we watch other people's visions flicker on a giant screen. As a professor tells a despondent college student in Matt Groening's comic strip *School Is Hell*, "The sooner you all face up to the fact that you are lazy, untalented losers, unfit to kiss the feet of a genius like Friedrich Nietzsche, the better off you'll be."

In many traditional cultures, art, like spirituality, saturates daily living. As the Balinese put it, "We have no art—everything we do is art." But in industrialized society, creativity, like so much else, has become compartmentalized, torn from the web of everyday life and assigned to specialists. Why should we paint, when we can buy a mass-produced print by a *real* artist that's much more attractive than anything we could come up with? Why blunder along on a musical instrument, when at the touch of a digital switch we can hear electronically enhanced world-class performances at any hour of day or night? In fact, why make anything of our lives at all, when we can watch ones with much more interesting scripts on TV?

Why? Because creativity, according to a growing number of people who have devoted their lives to exploring it, is an essential part of being human, a vital force without which we can exist, but not truly live. While many of us have become alienated from it, the damage is not irreversible, these artists say. In their rewriting of our cultural myth, creativity is depicted as an ongoing flow, within us and around us, that we can all open up to if we are willing to let down our guard.

As Stephen Nachmanovitch writes in *Free Play: Improvisation in Life and Art*, "What, then, is this seemingly endless stream of music, dance, imagery, acting, and speech that comes out of us whenever we let it? To some extent it is the stream of consciousness, a river of memories, fragments of melodies, emotions, fragrances, angers, old loves, fantasies. But we sense something else, beyond the personal, from a source that is both very old and very new. The raw material is a kind of flow—Heraclitus' river of time, or the great Tao, flowing through us, as us. . . . We can choose to tap into it or not to tap into it; we can find ourselves unwillingly opened up to it or unwillingly cut off from it. But it's always there."

In order to practice art as a means to awakening, it is essential to follow certain basic guidelines—all of which apply to life as surely as to art.

1. Trust your intuition. Whether you are writing, painting, singing, dancing, or just talking to a friend, it is crucial to honor your initial

In both the public and private spheres, we need innovative thinkers unfettered by "psycho-sclerosis," leaders with nimble minds tuned to high ideals and cosmic intelligence.

PHILIP GOLDBERG

impulses, the raw, uncensored vitality of your "first thoughts," which your internal critic will usually try to censor. Most of us have not been raised to honor our intuitions—on some deep level, we believe that if we do what we really want, disaster will inevitably ensue. In fact, sometimes our true desires are so deeply buried under a pile of "shoulds" that we don't even know what they are. "Creativity practice" is the ideal forum to learn to trust what happens if we allow ourselves to do exactly what we feel like doing.

2. Stay in the present. Forget about the painting you planned to paint, the great anecdote you wanted to tell, the rage you were feeling yesterday but can't quite whip up today. The wellspring of creativity is only accessible if you stay attuned to the here and now.

If you are terrified, express terror. If you are angry, let anger inform your creation. "You must always act on exactly what's going on," says performance artist Ruth Zaporah. "You can't try to be other than where you are. If we keep expressing what is, eventually that makes us acceptable to ourselves."

Boredom, says painter Michell Cassou, is a sure sign that you are not staying in the moment. "If you're bored, you're not doing what's coming to you. You're following an idea or a pattern, or maybe you think you should finish a painting the way you started it, or maybe you're trying to do a nice painting. You're manipulating the painting to do something you're not interested in doing."

3. Don't cross out. Don't erase what you have written, even if you have changed your mind. Don't paint over something you have done. If you are improvising with a partner, don't negate your partner's contributions but build on them, even if you don't like them. Commit yourself to your self-expressions. Create boldly, without caving in to afterthoughts and regret.

"This is the principle of respect," says Cassou. "If you're talking to me, and after every sentence I say 'You shouldn't have said that'—after a while you don't want to talk to me. It's the same thing with our intuition. If your intuition keeps giving you things and you keep telling it, "Hey, you made a mistake, let me fix it, let me change it,' it will stop talking to you."

"By crossing something out, or erasing something, or blocking

The goal of a creator—the way to the center—is his or her "work," whether it's teasing the solution to an important scientific problem like the structure of DNA or composing symphonies. The work—like the philosopher's stone—is the actual interface between the creator and the cosmos. Wholeness and truth must be manifest in the work for the creator to have accomplished the task.

JOHN BRIGGS

someone's expression, what you're saying is, 'I'm not open to the un-expected,'" says Zaporah. "This rule forces us to accept what's go-ing on over and over and over again until finally we don't want it any other way."

4. The process is what matters, not the product. Feeling empty in-side, we often want to reassure ourselves by creating something other people can admire. But what we are really hungering for, whether we know it or not, is a sense of aliveness, of deep contact with the sacred mystery of our lives.

If you want to draw a bird, you must become a bird.

HOKUSAI

The goal is not to produce a masterful painting, story, poem, song, or television script. The reason to create is the sheer pleasure and power of doing it, the vibrant aliveness that comes when we are contacting and expressing our true self. In this view, the product is simply a by-product, a relatively harmless side effect of the creative process. In the words of the *Bhagavad Gita*, we should perform our creative play "sacra-mentally, without attachment to results."

This purposeless, process-oriented approach is hard for most of us to accept because it contradicts all of our conditioning. "Most people only feel gratification when they look at what they've done. Sometimes people don't mind suffering for two hours on a painting, struggling, as long as they're going to like the result at the end," laments Cassou. "The beauty and interest and aliveness of the doing hasn't been valued in this society."

5. Don't analyze what you've done. This isn't psychotherapy, the art-ists all agree. It's not about examining the psychological significance of what you have created—it's about entering the flow of creativity. "Writing as therapy is like journal writing—there's a fascination with the emotions and the self. Writing as practice cuts through the emo-tions and takes you to an emptier place," says writer and Zen practi-tioner Natalie Goldberg.

"When you break a fence, you don't have to know what the fence is made of," agrees Cassou. "People paint an image and they want to know where it came from and what it means about them. They want to show it to people and ask them what they think about it. They make it so important, while for me the whole process is about not making impor-tant what comes out of you."

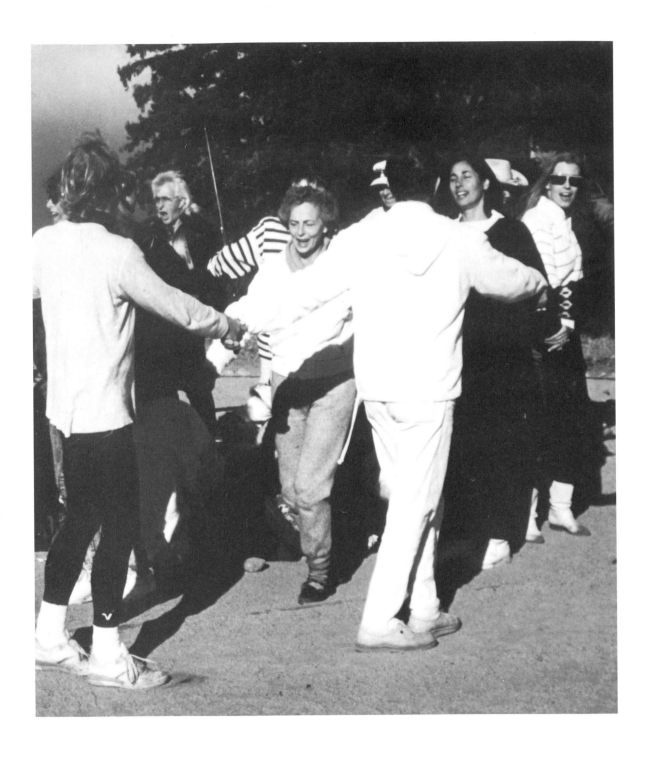

6. Special talent is not necessary. Tibetan Buddhist master Chogyam Trungpa once said, "There is no such thing as talent, only awareness." Or as Goldberg puts it, "If you connect with your own mind deep enough, it reverberates for everyone. That's what we call art."

It is not necessary to spend years acquiring technical skills before launching your own creations. In fact, an arsenal of painstakingly accumulated techniques can be a hindrance, because you will be tempted to rely on what you have learned, rather than reinventing your approach spontaneously, moment by moment.

"It's like trying to make a tree by gluing together branches, trunk, and leaves. Every part is right, but you can't do it," says Cassou. "But if you plant a seed, it might be growing slowly, but it breathes and lives."

7. Practice, practice, practice. Although you don't need talent, you do need perseverance, the courage to confront again and again the blank notebook, the empty canvas, the expectant eyes of the audience. The freedom with which you play must be balanced by the discipline with which you return, day after day, to the playground. Inspiration can only flow if you offer it a channel to flow through; spontaneity is only possible within structure.

The real goal is to live our lives as writing practice, as painting experience, as spontaneous song, as improvisational theater. Through honing the principles of art as practice, we can entrain our whole beings to the possibility of living by its guidelines. We can learn to contact the rest of our lives with passion and spontaneity, trusting our intuition, letting go of our preconceptions, inhibitions, plans, and judgments. Life, we begin to realize, *is* improvisation; the scene is constantly changing, defying our efforts to script it. We can learn to let go of the life we have already painted in our head, so we can work with the living, vibrant palette of the present.

It is frightening to let go into the unknown. But ultimately, it can give us a deeper security than we have ever had. "When the aliveness of creativity does not pass through you, it makes you old, however old you are," says Cassou. "I don't know how people can cope with all the pressures, all the demons, all the craziness of the world, if they don't have that contact. It gives you a solidity, a security. When you touch it, you have something that nobody can take from you. You have your root in your contact with the universe."

RESOURCES

Books

Aivanhov, O. M. *Creation: Artistic and Spiritual.* Frejus, France: Prosveta, 1987.

Briggs, J. *Fire in the Crucible: The Self-Creation of Creativity and Genius.* Los Angeles: J. P. Tarcher, 1990.

Cornell, J. *Drawing the Light from Within.* New York: Fireside/Simon Schuster, 1992.

Goldberg, N. *Wild Mind.* New York: Bantam, 1990.

————, *Writing Down the Bones.* Boston, MA: Shambhala, 1986.

Harman, W. *Higher Creativity: Liberating the Unconscious for Breakthrough Insights.* Los Angeles: J. P. Tarcher, 1984.

May, R. *The Courage to Create.* New York: Bantam, 1976.

Nachmanovitch, S. *Free Play: Improvisation in Life and Art.* Los Angeles: J. P. Tarcher, 1990.

Organizations

Action Theater (Ruth Zaporah), 1174 Cragmont Avenue, Berkeley, CA 94708. Tel.: (510) 841-9140.

Natalie Goldberg, P.O. Box 3014, Taos, NM 87571. Tel.: (505) 751-0430.

Music for People, RD 4, Box 221A, Keene, NH 03431. Tel.: (603) 352-4941.

The Painting Experience (Michell Cassou), 2101 20th Avenue, San Francisco, CA 94116. Tel.: (415) 564-8515.

PART SIX

THE PATH OF WISDOM: JNANA YOGA

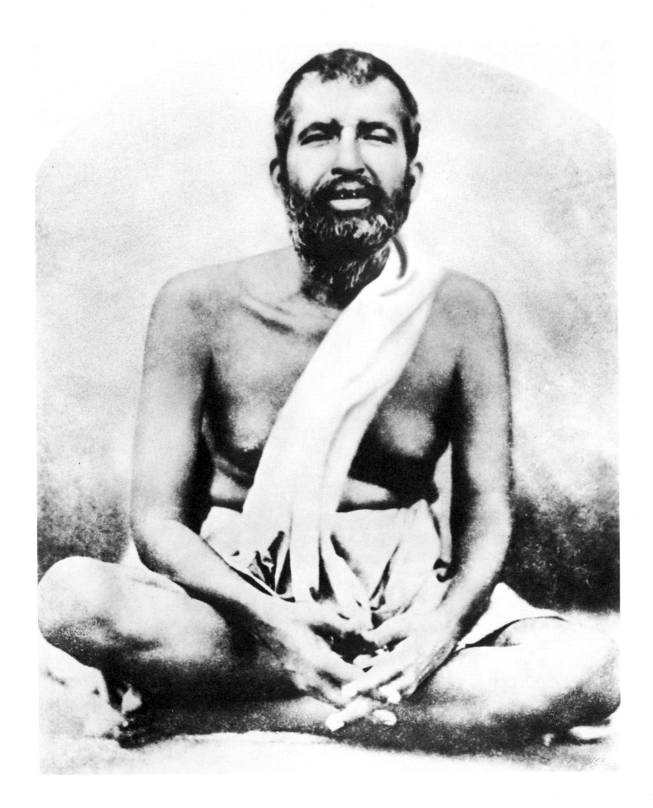

THIRTEEN

Insight Is Liberating

The yoga masters of bygone ages developed a variety of approaches to cater to the individual needs of different personality types. Jnana yoga is for the person who is capable of exercising considerable discernment in all matters. To be sure, this is not the path of intellectuals, who are best advised to cultivate the power of the open heart. The kind of intelligence called for on the path of jnana yoga is not that of ordinary learning, but a higher sensitivity that renders life more transparent. It is a form of wisdom, and jnana yoga seeks to foster that wisdom—until it flowers into the fullness of Self-realization. This chapter introduces four great masters of jnana yoga, two from India and two from Western countries: Ramana Maharshi, Nisargadatta Maharaj, Jean Klein, and Paul Brunton.

The paths of knowledge are countless, and the windows of light are innumerable.

BEINSA DOUNO
(PETER DEUNOV)

FROM THE UNREAL TO THE REAL

"Lead us from the unreal to the real, from falsehood to truth, from darkness to light." This ancient Hindu prayer expresses a core sentiment that is universal among spiritual seekers. But what is meant by "real" and "unreal"? For the yogi, only the Divine, the Self, is overwhelmingly real. All else is, if not illusory, in some way less real or unreal. Western students of yoga are often confused about this philosophical point, which, in the final analysis, is not a theoretical problem at all, but a matter of firsthand experience.

The yogi who has traveled the spiritual path to the end enjoys a

A yogi free from yoga and non-yoga, or a worldly man free from enjoyment or non-enjoyment: thus he walks leisurely, filled with his mind's innate bliss.

AVADHUTA GITA VII.9

view of existence that is entirely different from our ordinary everyday experience. We normally experience the world as if it existed outside us and as if it were constituted of countless separate objects, which we, as the subject, confront. Our eyes serve as windows onto that external world populated by innumerable beings and things. For the enlightened adept, however, subject and object are not divorced from one another, and the world is a seamless continuum. This is the perennial wisdom of nonduality (advaita), as taught by the adepts of jnana yoga.

The yogic perspective has the distinct advantage of conforming to the latest discoveries of modern physics, whereas our ordinary perception of the world is clearly pre-Einsteinian. Moreover, for countless generations the great adepts of the world's spiritual traditions have been speaking, writing, and singing about that suprasensuous, mind-transcending continuum, as being not only supremely conscious but also unimaginably blissful.

The Hindus call it *brahman*, when viewed as the foundation of the world of our senses, and *atman*, when regarded as the very center of our subjective existence. There is no actual difference between brahman and atman. When we realize the atman, our inmost Self, we also realize brahman, the ultimate basis of the objective world.

From the vantage-point of that realization, the world as it appears to the unenlightened person is indeed less real. The Hindu sages like to compare it to a dream landscape. When we awaken from the dream, we know we have been dreaming, but while we are immersed in the dream experience we absolutely believe the unfolding drama. The Self-realized sage no longer believes the dreamlike drama that all unenlightened beings find so compelling.

The world as it is experienced through the five senses is not entirely unreal in itself, only our perception of it is extremely limited. It is so limited, in fact, that by comparison with the sage's view of the world as an unbroken continuum, it appears to be an unfortunate distortion.

The yogi's work consists in jettisoning, step by step, all misconceptions about existence and "remembering" that which is real—the Self, or Divine. The many techniques and practices of the yogic path are designed to assist us in expanding our perception of the world. Especially through concentration and meditation, we learn that the world is not as solid as we like to believe, but a vast field of energy. As we acquire the ability to sense and consciously interact with that field of energy, we are gradually guided, through layer after layer, to its utmost limit.

Beyond that final perimeter, we discover our "true original face"—
the Self.

In the course of our efforts, we cultivate the capacity for ever more
acute discernment (viveka) between the Self and the many substitute
realities that we perceive as long as our ego-personality serves as the
focal point for our perceptions. The ego obliges us to see everything in
perspective, but perspective is not a quality that is inherent in what is
seen. It is a function of the human mind by which we carve out a con-
veniently small slice of reality so that we can grasp it.

Upon enlightenment, the ego is transcended and so are its pecu-
liarly limiting perspectives. The sage's "vision" is a 360-degree pano-
ramic view, which takes in all space and all time. This is possible only
because the sage *is* everything that he perceives. *Aham brahma asmi*, "I am
the Absolute." This classic mystical proclamation is not mere metaphor.
The enlightened being has in effect slipped out of the world of space
and time. His body-mind will continue to exist and age, but the sage is
no longer identifying with that limited manifestation. He is infinite and
blissful, regardless of the sensations that run through his body or the
thoughts that pop into his mind.

If we find this state puzzling, then we must marvel no less about
our own paradoxical condition. For, even though we believe the dream
of our unenlightened existence, we are yet eternally free and no less
blissful than the sage. But this truth is for us to discover and for the sage
to celebrate.

*Subject and object are only one.
The barrier between them cannot
be said to have broken down as a
result of recent experience in the
physical sciences, for this barrier
does not exist.*

ERWIN SCHROEDINGER

RESOURCES

Books

Aivanhov, O. M. *The Path of Silence*. Frejus, France: Prosveta, 1990. Distributed by Prosveta U.S.A., Los Angeles.

Brunton, P. *Enlightened Mind, Divine Mind*. Burdett, NY: Larson Publications, 1988.

Deane, D. *Wisdom, Bliss and Common Sense: Secrets of Self-Transformation*.
Wheaton, IL: Quest Books, 1989.

Frawley, D. *Beyond the Mind*. Salt Lake City, UT: Passage Press, 1992.

Swami Vivekananda. *Jnana Yoga*. New York: Ramakrishna-Vivekananda
Center, 1982.

BE WHO YOU ARE:
AN INTERVIEW WITH JEAN KLEIN
BY STEPHAN BODIAN

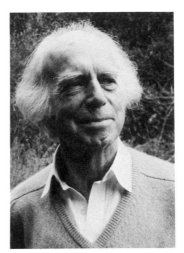

JEAN KLEIN

Jean Klein is a contemporary master of Advaita Vedanta, the philosophical culmination of the Hindu tradition. According to this nondualist teaching, the entire universe is, in essence, a single reality—Consciousness, the true Self of all beings—to which each of us is inherently capable of awakening.

In person, Jean Klein has the vigor, freshness, and attentive curiosity of a child. He speaks English slowly, with an accent that blends his native Czech, the German of his school days, and the French he has spoken in France and Switzerland since before the war. Of his background he talks little, believing it to be of no importance in the critical work of realizing our true nature.

Klein is unpretentious. If one weren't aware that he was a master of Advaita, one might just as easily mistake him, on first meeting, for the old shopkeeper down the street—sweet, a little eccentric, with a spark of some secret wisdom in his eyes. Although he has been teaching for nearly 30 years, Klein has established no centers or organizations. Instead, he prefers to travel from place to place answering questions and teaching his special brand of hatha yoga to those who gather, in six European countries and the United States, to study with him.

What about the whole notion of the spiritual path—the idea that you enter a path, follow a certain prescribed way of practice, and eventually achieve some goal?

It belongs to psychology, to the realm of the mind. These are sweets for the mind.

What about the argument that if you don't practice, you can't attain anything?

You must first see that in all practice you project a goal, a result. And in projecting a result you remain constantly in the representation of what you project. What you *are* fundamentally is a natural giving up. When the mind becomes clear, there is a giving up, a stillness, fulfilled with a current of love. As long as there's a meditator, there's no meditation. When the meditator disappears, there is meditation.

So by practicing some meditation technique, you are somehow interfering with that giving up.

Absolutely.

How?

You interfere because you think there is something to attain. But in reality what you *are* fundamentally is nothing to obtain, nothing to achieve. You can only achieve something that remains in the mind, knowledge. You must see the difference. Being yourself has nothing to do with accumulating knowledge.

In certain traditions—Zen, for one—you have to meditate in order to exhaust the mind; through meditating, the mind eventually wears itself out and comes to rest. Then a kind of opening takes place. But you're suggesting that the process of meditating somehow gets in the way of this opening.

Yes. This practicing is still produced by will. For me, the point of meditation is only to look for the meditator. When we find out that the meditator, the one who looks for God, for beauty, for peace, is only a product of the brain and that there is therefore nothing to find, there is a giving up. What remains is a current of silence. You can never come to this silence through practice, through achievement. Enlightenment—being understanding—is instantaneous.

Once you've attained this enlightenment or this current, do you then exist in it all the time?

Constantly. But it's not a state. When there's a state, there is mind.

So in the midst of this current there is also activity?

Oh, yes. Activity and non-activity. Timeless awareness is the life behind all activity and non-activity. Activity and non-activity are more or less superimpositions upon this constant beingness. It is behind the three states of waking, dreaming, and sleeping, beyond inhalation and exhalation. Of course, the words "beyond" and "behind" have a spatial connotation that does not belong to this beingness.

In the midst of all activity, then, you are aware of this presence, this clarity.

Yes, "presence" is a good word. You *are* presence, but you are not aware of it.

You've often called what you teach the direct way, and you've contrasted it with what you call progressive teachings, including the classical yoga tradition and most

We would not be satisfied with a merely conceptualized God, because when the concept slips away, that God also vanishes. Rather we should have the essential God who is exalted far above human thoughts or any creature. Such a God does not vanish, unless a person deliberately turns away from Him.

MEISTER ECKHART

Those who have had the good fortune to live in close proximity with a saint or realized person have all testified to the intense atmosphere of peace which radiates out from them to a great distance into the surroundings.

JACK SANTA MARIA

forms of Buddhism. *What is the danger of progressive teachings, and why do you think the direct way is closer to the truth?*

In the progressive way, you use various techniques and gradually attain higher and higher states. But you remain constantly in the mind, in the subject-object relationship. Even when you give up the last object, you still remain in the duality of subject and object. You are still in a kind of blank state, and this blank state itself becomes an extremely subtle object. In this state, it is very difficult to give up the subject-object relationship. Once you've attained it, you're locked into it, fixed to it. There's a kind of quietness, but there's no flavor, no taste.

You say that any kind of practice is a hindrance, but at the same time you suggest practices to people. You teach a form of yoga to your students, and to some you recommend self-inquiry, such as the question, "Who am I?" It sounds paradoxical—no practice, but you teach a practice. What practices do you teach, and why do you use practices at all?

To try to practice and to try not to practice are both practice. I would rather say listen, be attentive, and see that you really are *not* attentive. When you see in certain moments in daily life that you are not attentive, in those moments you are attentive. Then see how you function. That is very important. Be completely objective. Don't judge, compare, criticize, evaluate. Become more and more accustomed to listening. Listen to your body, without judging, without reference—just listen. Listen to all the situations in daily life. Listen from the whole mind, not from a mind divided by positive and negative. Look from the whole, the global. Students generally observe that most of the time they are not in this listening, although our natural way of behavior is listening.

The path you are describing is often called the "high path with no railing," which is the most difficult path of all. The average person wouldn't know where to begin to do what you're talking about. Most could probably be attentive to their inattention, but after that, what? There's nothing to grasp onto.

No, there's nothing to grasp, nothing to find. But it is only apparently a difficult path; actually, I would say it is the easiest path.

The thought self, the emotion self, the action self, and the observing self are complementary phases of consciousness; they are not the fundamental source of individual being. That source is beyond ordinary awareness; mystics call it the Self or Truth or Knowledge.

ARTHUR J. DEIKMAN

How so?

Listening to something is easy because it doesn't go through the mind. It is our natural behavior. Evaluation, comparison, is very difficult because it involves mental effort. In this listening there's a welcoming of all that happens, an unfolding, and this unfolding, this welcoming, is timeless. All that you welcome appears in this timelessness, and there's a moment when you feel yourself timeless, feel yourself in welcoming, feel yourself in listening, in attention. Because attention has its own taste, its own flavor. There's attention to something, but there's also attention in which there's no object: nothing to see, nothing to hear, nothing to touch, only attention.

And in that moment of pure attention, you realize the one who's being attentive?

I would say that this attention, completely free from choice and reflection, refers to itself. Because it is essentially timeless.

The Zen master Dogen said: "Take the backward step that turns your light inwardly to illuminate the self." That seems to be similar to what you are talking about.

Yes, but one must be careful. Turning the head inward is still doing something. And there's really no inward and no outward.

I notice that you use the word "attention." Is this the same as what the Buddhists call mindfulness—being acutely aware of every movement, every sensation, every thought?

Mindfulness mainly emphasizes the object, the perceived, and not the perceiving, which can never be an object, just as the eye can never see its seeing. The attention I'm speaking of is objectless, directionless, and in it all that is perceived exists potentially. Mindfulness implies a subject-object relation, but attention is non-dual. Mindfulness is intentional; attention is the real state of the mind, free from volition.

What about the yoga you teach, which you call "body-work"? What is it, and why do you teach it?

You are not your body, senses, and mind; body, senses, and mind are expressions of your timeless awareness. But to completely under-

Brahman is not a particular experience, level of consciousness or state of soul—rather it is precisely whatever level you happen to have now, and realizing this confers upon one a profound center of peace that underlies and persists throughout the worst depressions, anxieties, and fears.

KEN WILBER

Realizing that I am the center of the universe makes it easy for me to realize that you are too, and that there are space and time enough for you and me and all other beings.

GEORGE LEONARD

Incarnated in a great teacher, great ideas become pure energy and love—the teacher acts and lives the ideas; they are his being.

JACOB NEEDLEMAN

stand that you are not something, you must first see what you are not. You cannot say "I am not the body" without knowing what it is. So you inquire, you explore, you look, you listen. And you discover that you know only certain fractions of your body, certain sensations, and these are more or less reactions, resistance. Eventually you come to a body feeling that you have never had before, because when you listen it unfolds, and the sensitive body, the energy body, appears. It is most important to feel and come into contact with the energy body. Because in the beginning your body is more or less a pattern or superficial structure in the mind, made up of reactions and resistance. But when you really listen to the body, you are no longer an accomplice to these reactions, and the body comes to its natural feeling, which is emptiness.

The real body in its original state is emptiness, a completely vacant state. Then you feel the appearance of the elastic body, which is the energy body. When we speak of "body-work," it is mainly to find this energy body. Once the energy body has been experienced, the physical body works completely differently. The muscle structure, the skin, the flesh, is seen and felt in a completely new way. Even the muscles and bones function differently.

RESOURCES

Books

Klein, J. *I Am*. Santa Barbara, CA: Third Millennium, 1990.

_____. *The Transmission of the Flame*. Santa Barbara, CA: Third Millennium, 1991.

_____. *Who Am I?* London: Element Books, 1988.

Organizations

Jean Klein Foundation, P.O. Box 940, Larkspur, CA 94939. The Foundation provides information on upcoming events and available publications by Jean Klein.

WHO AM I?
BY RAMANA MAHARSHI

The following essay, reproduced here only in part, was written at the turn of the century. Although Sri Ramana was then only a young man in his early twenties, his Self-realization was as solid as his favorite mountain, Arunachala, in South India where he spent most of his life.

Every living being longs always to be happy, untainted by sorrow; and everyone has the greatest love for himself, which is solely due to the fact that happiness is his real nature. Hence, in order to realize that inherent and untainted happiness, which indeed he daily experiences when the mind is subdued in deep sleep, it is essential that he should know himself. For obtaining such knowledge the enquiry "Who am I?" in quest of the Self is the best means.

"Who am I?" I am not this physical body, nor am I the five organs of sense perception; I am not the five organs of external activity, nor am I the five vital forces, nor am I even the thinking mind. Neither am I that unconscious state of nescience which retains merely the subtle vasanas (latencies of the mind), while being free from the functional activity of the sense-organs and of the mind, and being unaware of the existence of the objects of sense-perception.

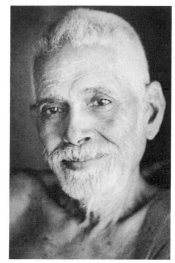

RAMANA MAHARSHI

Therefore, summarily rejecting all the above-mentioned physical adjuncts and their functions, saying "I am not this; no, nor am I this, nor this"—that which then remains separate and alone by itself, that pure Awareness is what I am. This Awareness is by its very nature Sat-Chit-Ananda (Existence-Consciousness-Bliss). . . .

By a steady and continuous investigation into the nature of the mind, the mind is transformed into *That* to which the "I" refers; and that is in fact the Self. Mind has necessarily to depend for its existence on something gross; it never subsists by itself. It is this mind that is otherwise called the subtle body, ego, jiva, or soul.

That which arises in the physical body as "I" is the mind. If one enquires whence the "I"-thought in the body arises in the first instance, it will be found that it is from hrdayam, or the Heart. That is the source and stay of the mind. Or again, even if one merely continuously repeats to oneself inwardly "I-I" with the entire mind fixed thereon, that also leads one to the same source.

The first and foremost of all the thoughts that arise in the mind is the primal "I"-thought. It is only after the rise or origin of the "I"-thought that innumerable other thoughts arise. In other words, only after the first personal pronoun, "I," has arisen, do the second and third personal pronouns ("you, he," etc.) occur to the mind; and they cannot subsist without the former.

Since every other thought can occur only after the rise of the

"I"-thought and since the mind is nothing but a bundle of thoughts, it is only through the enquiry "Who am I?" that the mind subsides. Moreover, the integral "I"-thought, implicit in such enquiry, having destroyed all other thoughts, gets itself finally destroyed or consumed, just as the stick used for stirring the burning funeral pyre gets consumed.

Even when extraneous thoughts sprout up during such enquiry, do not seek to complete the rising thought, but instead, deeply enquire within, "To whom has this thought occurred?" No matter how many thoughts thus occur to you, if you would with acute vigilance enquire immediately as and when each individual thought arises to whom it has occurred, you would find it is to "me." If then you enquire "Who am I?" the mind gets introverted and the rising thought also subsides. In this manner as you persevere more and more in the practice of Self-enquiry, the mind acquires increasing strength and power to abide in its Source. . . .

This state of mere inherence in pure Being is known as the Vision of Wisdom. Such inherence means and implies the entire subsidence of the mind in the Self. Nothing other than this and no psychic powers of the mind, such as thought-reading, telepathy and clairvoyance, can be Wisdom.

Atman alone exists and is real. The threefold reality of world, individual soul, and God is, like the illusory appearance of silver in the mother of pearl, an imaginary creation in the Atman. They appear and disappear simultaneously. The Self alone is the world, the "I" and God. All that exists is but the manifestation of the Supreme. . . .

That which is Bliss is also the Self. Bliss and the Self are not distinct and separate but are one and the same. And *That* alone is real. In no single one of the countless objects of the mundane world is there anything that can be called happiness. It is through sheer ignorance and unwisdom that we fancy that happiness is obtained from them. On the contrary, when the mind is externalized, it suffers pain and anguish. The truth is that every time our desires get fulfilled, the mind, turning to its source, experiences only that happiness which is natural to the Self. . . .

If the ego rises, all else will also rise; if it subsides, all else will also subside. The deeper the humility with which we conduct ourselves, the better it is for us. If only the mind is kept under control, what matters it where one may happen to be?

A mind that has had super-conscious experience needs no inference or logic to understand the existence of God.

SWAMI AKHILANANDA

All our words about God are metaphorical rather than literal statements. They function well as pointers aiming us toward the Goy beyond the words, or as vessels welcoming us to encounter God between the lines. Even the most hallowed formulation becomes idolatrous if we mistake the name for the Reality toward whom the name leads. . . .
Although God is One, no one image or title is adequate.

GENIA PAULI HADDON

RESOURCES

Books

Lakshman, S. K. *Maha Yoga; or, The Upanishadic Lore in the Light of the Teachings of Bhagavan Sri Ramana.* Tiruvannamalai, India: Venkataraman, 1967.

Osborne, A., ed. *The Collected Works of Ramana Maharshi.* New York: Weiser, 1970.

————. *The Teachings of Ramana Maharshi.* New York: Samuel Weiser, 1978.

Periodicals

The Mountain Path, a quarterly journal, is dedicated to the philosophy of Vedanta and to keeping the memory of Sri Ramana alive. Subscription address: Sri Ramanasramam, P.O. Tiruvannamalai, 606 603, South India.

Pathways. This is a quarterly publication which seeks to provide a forum for the interchange of spiritual and philosophical ideals. It is published by the Ramana Maharshi Foundation of America. There is no subscription at present, but donations are welcome.

Organizations

Ramana Maharshi Foundation of America. Publisher of *Pathways* 5222 Lake Village Drive, Sarasota, FL 34235.

THE TIMELESS WISDOM OF NONDUALITY: SAYINGS BY NISARGADATTA MAHARAJ
BY ROBERT POWELL, PH.D.

Nisargadatta Maharaj (1897–1981) was a Self-realized adept who, like Sri Ramana Maharshi, taught the simple but profound truths of jnana yoga to anyone who cared to climb the steps to his small room on the second floor of his house in the middle of Bombay.

■ ■ ■

Awareness becomes consciousness when it has an object. The object changes all the time. In consciousness there is movement; awareness by itself is motionless and timeless, here and now.

Names and shapes change incessantly. Know yourself to be the changeless witness of the changeful mind. That is enough.

Your own self is your ultimate teacher. The outer teacher is merely a milestone. It is only your inner teacher that will walk with you to the goal, for he *is* that goal.

Life goes on, soul goes on, purpose goes on, reality goes on. Immortality is inevitable.

MANLY PALMER HALL

My experience is that everything is bliss. But the desire for bliss creates pain. Thus bliss becomes the seed of pain. The entire universe of pain is born of desire. Give up the desire for pleasure and you will not even know what pain is.

Nobody ever fails in Yoga. . . . It is slow in the beginning and rapid in the end. When one is fully matured, realization is explosive.

Wisdom is eternally negating the unreal. To see the unreal is wisdom. Beyond this lies the inexpressible.

The pure mind sees things as they are—bubbles in consciousness. These bubbles are appearing, disappearing and reappearing, without having real being. No particular cause can be ascribed to them, for each is caused by all and affects all. Each bubble is a body and all these bodies are mine.

The moment you know your real being, you are afraid of nothing. Death gives freedom and power. To be free in the world, you must die to the world. Then the universe is your own, it becomes your body, an expression and a tool. The happiness of being absolutely free is beyond description. On the other hand, he who is afraid of freedom cannot die.

Learn to look without imagination, to listen without distortion: that is all. Stop attributing names and shapes to the essentially nameless and formless, realize that every mode of perception is subjective, that what is seen or heard, touched or smelled, felt or thought, expected or imagined, is in the mind and not in reality, and you will experience peace and freedom from fear.

The mind creates time and space, and takes its own creations for reality. All is here and now, but we do not see it. Truly, all is in me and by me. There is nothing else. The very idea of "else" is a disaster and a calamity.

Just keep in mind the feeling "I am," merge in it, until your mind and feeling become one. By repeated attempts you will stumble on the right balance of attention and affection, and your mind will be firmly established in the thought-feeling "I am." Whatever you think, say, or do, this sense of immutable and affectionate being remains as the ever-present background of the mind.

To deal with things, knowledge of things is needed. To deal with people, you need insight, sympathy. To deal with yourself, you need nothing. Be what you are—conscious being—and don't stray away from yourself.

We are all pilgrim people on our way toward wholeness and fullness of life.

ELAINE V. EMTH AND
JANET H. GREENHUT

RESOURCES

Books

Dunn, J., ed. *Seeds of Consciousness: The Wisdom of Sri Nisargadatta Maharaj.* Durham, NC: Acorn Press, 1985.

Powell, R., ed. *The Nectar of the Lord's Feet: Final Teachings of Sri Nisargadatta Maharaj.* Longmead, England: Element Books, 1987.

————. *The Wisdom of Sri Nisargadatta Maharaj.* Yorktown, NY: Globe Press Books, 1992.

THE SPONTANEOUS LIFE OF ENLIGHTENMENT
BY PAUL BRUNTON

British writer Paul Brunton (1898–1981) traveled widely in the East and had many memorable encounters with great sages. His first book, *A Search in Secret India* (1934), introduced Sri Ramana Maharshi to the West. In subsequent years, the sagely Brunton showed an exemplary dedication to the perennial philosophy of nonduality. His experience and wisdom is distilled in his many books, but especially his posthumously published *Notebooks.*

■ ■ ■

Ramana Maharshi often used the term *sahaja samadhi* to describe what he regarded as the best state. Although the word *samadhi* is too often associated with yogic trance, there is nothing of the kind in his

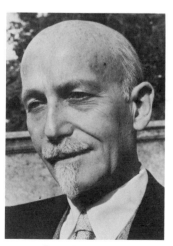

PAUL BRUNTON   269

use of the term. He said it was the best state because it was quite natural, nothing forced, artificial, or temporary. We may equate it with Zen's "This life is very life" and "Walk On!"

Sahaja samadhi is not broken into intervals, is permanent, and involves no special effort. Its arisal is instantaneous and without progressive stages. It can accompany daily activity without interfering with it. It is a settled calm and complete inner quiet.

There are no distinguishing marks that an outside observer can use to identify a *sahaja*-conscious man because *sahaja* represents consciousness itself rather than its transitory states.

Sahaja has been called the lightning flash. Philosophy considers it to be the most desirable goal.

This is illustrated with a classic instance of Indian spirituality involving a king named Janaka. One day he was about to mount his horse and put one foot into the stirrup which hung from the saddle. As he was about to lift himself upwards into the saddle, the "lightning flash" struck his consciousness. He was instantly carried away and concentrated so deeply that he failed for some time to lift himself up any higher. From that day onwards he lived in *sahaja samadhi* which was always present within him.

Those at the state of achieved *sahaja* are under no compulsion to continue to meditate any more or to practise yoga. They often do—either because of inclinations produced by past habits or as a means of helping other persons. In either case it is experienced as a pleasure. Because this consciousness is permanent, the experiencer does not need to go into meditation. This is despite the outward appearance of a person who places himself in the posture of meditation in order to achieve something.

What is the difference between the state of deepest contemplation which the Hindus call *nirvikalpa samadhi*, and that which they call *sahaja samadhi*? The first is only a temporary experience, that is, it begins and ends but the man actually experiences an uplift of consciousness, he gains a new and higher outlook. But *sahaja* is continuous unbroken realization that as Overself [transcendental Self] he always was, is, and shall be. It is not a feeling that something new and higher has been gained. What is the absolute test which distinguishes one condition from the other, since both are awareness of the Overself? In *nirvikalpa* the ego vanishes but reappears when the ordinary state is resumed:

When we pour a drop of water into the turbulent ocean, then that drop is transmuted into the ocean, not the ocean into the drop. The same occurs with the soul: When God withdraws the soul into Himself, then it is transmuted into Him, so that the soul becomes divine rather than God becomes the soul.

MEISTER ECKHART

hence it has only been lulled, even though it has been slightly weakened by the process. In *sahaja* the ego is rooted out once and for all! It not only vanishes, but it cannot reappear.

RESOURCES

Books

Brunton, P. *The Hidden Teaching Beyond Yoga*. York Beach, MN: Samuel Weiser, 1984.

————. *The Notebooks of Paul Brunton*. 16 vols. Burdett, NY: Larson Publications, 1984–1988.

————. *A Search in Secret India*. York Beach, MN: Samuel Weiser, 1985.

Hurst, K. T. *Paul Brunton: A Personal View*. Burdett, NY: Larson Publications, 1989. The only biography of Brunton.

Standing on the bare ground— my head bathed by the blithe air, and uplifted into infinite space— all mean egotism vanishes. I become a transparent eye-ball; I am nothing; I see all; the currents of the Universal Being circulate through me; I am part or parcel of God.

RALPH WALDO EMERSON

About the Contributors

Omraam Mikhael Aivanhov was a Bulgarian-born spiritual teacher, who taught in France for nearly fifty years until his death in 1986. While he did not write any books, his numerous talks are being published by Prosveta. Over forty titles have so far been translated into English.

Renee Beck is a Universal Life minister, director of counseling at Contra Costa Alternative High School, and a licensed marriage, family and child therapist working in Oakland, California. She is also co-author of *The Art of Ritual.*

Joan Borysenko, Ph.D., is a cell biologist and co-founder of the Mind/ Body Clinic at New England Deaconess Hospital, Harvard Medical School. She is the author of the bestseller *Minding the Body, Mending the Mind* and *Guilt Is the Teacher, Love Is the Lesson.*

Paul Brunton, who died in 1983, was a journalist turned sage. His many publications paved the way for Eastern wisdom in the West. Among his best known books are *A Search in Secret India, The Hidden Teaching Beyond Yoga,* and *The Secret Path.* His notebooks have been published in 16 volumes.

Diana Leafe Christian is a former book review editor of *Yoga Journal* and current research editor of *The Earth Changes Report* newsletter.

Anne Cushman is an associate editor of *Yoga Journal* and contributes articles to that magazine and other publications.

Ram Dass, who was born Richard Alpert, is one of the popular heroes of the American counter-culture of the sixties. He has authored many books, including *Be Here Now, Grist for the Mill, Journey of Awakening,* and *Compassion in Action.* His primary work is with the Seva Foundation, an international community dedicated to compassionate action.

Larry Dossey, M.D., is well known for his insightful books on the interface between medicine and avant-garde science and culture. His works include *Space, Time, and Medicine* and *The Meaning of Medicine.*

Ken Dychtwald, Ph.D., is a leading figure in the holistic health field and president of Age Wave, Inc., an education and communications firm. He is the author of several books, including *Bodymind* and *Age Wave.*

Donna Farhi, formerly Donna Farhi Schuster, is a certified Iyengar yoga teacher and educational bodywork therapist practicing in the San Francisco Bay Area. She regularly contributes articles to *Yoga Journal.*

Peggy R. Gillispie is a freelance writer. She was the assistant director of the Stress Reduction Department at University of Massachusetts Medical Center and is the co-author of *Less Stress in 30 Days* (Signet). She has led workshops throughout the U.S. and currently works at the Belchertown Wellness Center in Massachusetts.

S. N. Goenka is a renowned Burmese meditation master who lives in India. He is the spiritual head of the Vipassana International Academy in Igatpuri, near Bombay, an organization that has branches in countries around the world.

Daniel Goleman, Ph.D., is a former senior editor of *Psychology Today* and the author of *The Meditative Mind* and *Vital Lies, Simple Truths.*

Ken Keyes, Jr. is the author of a number of books, including the bestsellers *The Hundredth Monkey* and *Handbook to Higher Consciousness.* He lives and works at the Ken Keyes College in Coos Bay, Oregon.

Jean Klein teaches Advaita Vedanta in Europe and the United States. Some of his talks have been published in book form, notably *Who Am I?* and *I Am.*

Tanya Kucak is an herbalist, writer, and editor who travels between the Pacific coast and the Southwest deserts.

Judith Lasater, Ph.D., graduated in East-West psychology and is a registered physical therapist. A student of B. K. S. Iyengar, she teaches yoga at the Iyengar Yoga Institute in San Francisco.

Hart Lazer teaches Iyengar yoga at the Yoga Center in Winnipeg, Canada.

Joel Levey, Ph.D., and **Michelle Levey,** M.A., are co-founders of InnerWork Technologies, Inc., a Seattle-based company that builds synergy between personal and organizational transformation. They are co-authors of *Quality of Mind* and *The Fine Arts of Relaxation, Concentration, Meditation.*

Jane MacMullen is a long-time practitioner of yoga and a holistic health practitioner.

Joanna Macy is a teacher of world religions and an activist for peace and justice. She travels worldwide to give lectures and workshops on psychological and spiritual resources for effective social action. She also is the author of *Despair and Personal Power in the Nuclear Age* and *World as Lover, World As Self.*

D. Patrick Miller is a writer who publishes widely in the journalism of consciousness. He is a senior writer of *Yoga Journal.*

Elise Browning Miller is a teacher of Iyengar yoga at the California Yoga Center in Palo Alto, specializing in remedial yoga for scoliosis and back pain sufferers.

Richard C. Miller, Ph.D. is director of The Marin School of Yoga in Mill Valley, California, and a founding member of Viniyoga America. He also maintains a private practice in psychotherapy, hypnotherapy, and yoga therapy.

Victoria Moran is a writer and practitioner of yoga and the author of *Compassion, the Ultimate Ethic* and *The Love-Powered Diet.*

Donald Moyer has studied hatha yoga since 1972, primarily with B. K. S. Iyengar and Prashant Iyengar, and is director of the Yoga Room in Berkeley, California. He also is a co-director of Rodmell Press and regularly contributes articles to *Yoga Journal.*

Jacob Needleman, Ph.D., is a professor of philosophy at San Francisco State University and is well-known as the author of many books, including *The Heart of Philosophy, The New Religions,* and *Money and the Meaning of Life.*

Gretchen Rose Newmark, M.A., is a registered dietitian in private practice in Santa Monica, California.

Nisargadatta Maharaj was a merchant in Bombay who had realized the Self. Until his death in 1981, he instructed anyone who cared to come to his home in the wisdom of Advaita Vedanta.

Ramana Maharshi, who died in 1955, was one of the great contemporary masters of Advaita Vedanta. For over thirty years he lived at Arunachala mountain near Madras, India.

Peace Pilgrim, one of the spiritual giants of contemporary America, covered tens of thousands of miles in her twenty-eight-year pilgrimage for peace. She died in 1981.

Mary Pullig Schatz, M.D., is the author of *Back Care Basics: A Doctor's Gentle Yoga Program for Back and Neck Pain Relief* (Rodmell Press, Berkeley, Calif.). A certified Iyengar yoga teacher in Nashville, Tennessee, she teaches yoga to health professionals, medical patients and other yoga teachers. She is a regular contributor to *Yoga Journal* and *The Physician and Sportsmedicine* and serves on the editorial board of both magazines.

John Seed is the founder and director of the Rainforest Information center, in New South Wales, Australia. He organizes conferences on deep ecology, meditation, and social action and is the co-producer of the film "Earth First," and co-author of *Thinking Like a Mountain.*

Carolyn R. Shaffer is a writer and workshop leader in Berkeley, California. She is co-author of *Creating Community Anywhere.*

Gary Snyder is a Pulitzer-prize-winning poet and the author of many books, including *The Old Ways* and *Passage Through India.*

Stuart Sovatsky, Ph.D., is a psychotherapist in private practice in Oakland, California. He is also director of the Kundalini Clinic for Counseling and Research, and has studied yoga and meditation with various teachers. He is the author of *Passions of Innocence.*

Karen Turner, M.A., is a writer and psychotherapist in Marin County, California, and specializes in midlife transitions and spiritual awakening.

Frances Vaughan, Ph.D., a psychologist practicing in Mill Valley, California, is the author of *Awakening Intuition* and *The Inward Arc,* and co-editor of *Beyond Ego.*

Swami Vivekananda, the principal disciple of Sri Ramakrishna, was one of the earliest promulgators of yoga wisdom in the West. He made his debut as a spiritual leader at the 1893 Parliament of Religions in Chicago. He died in 1902 at the age of thirty-nine.

Thich Nhat Hanh is a Vietnamese Buddhist monk who lectures widely and holds meditation retreats in North America and Europe. He is the author of over sixty books in English and Vietnamese, including *Being Peace* and *Peace Is Every Step*.

John Welwood, Ph.D. is a clinical psychologist and psychotherapist in private practice. His books include *Awakening the Heart, Challenge of the Heart,* and *Journey of the Heart*.

Ken Wilber is a leading theoretician in the field of transpersonal psychology. His widely read books include *The Spectrum of Consciousness, The Atman Project,* and *Up From Eden*.

Bryan Wittine, Ph.D., is a psychotherapist in private practice in Oakland, California, and co-founder and former director of the Transpersonal Counseling Psychology program at John F. Kennedy University.

COPYRIGHTS AND PERMISSIONS

page 243; Fred Stimson, page 26; Ray Stott/The Image Works, page 148; Clark Thomas/Nashville, pages 87, 89, 90; Lawrence Watson, pages 58, 62; Courtesy Yoga Centre Winnipeg, pages xiv, 46; Courtesy Zen Center of Los Angeles, page 177.

Every effort has been made to contact the sources of the articles in this book. All articles printed by permission of the authors unless otherwise noted.

"A Nonviolent Approach to Extending Your Limits" from *Bodymind* by Ken Dychtwald, published by Jeremy P. Tarcher, Inc. Reprinted by permission of the author.

"The Yoga of Eating," from *Yoga of Nutrition* by Omraam Mikhael Aivanhov. Copyright by Editions Prosueta, SA Fréjus, France. Reprinted by permission of Editions Prosueta, SA Fréjus, France.

"Turning Stress into Strength," from *Quality of Mind: Tools for Self-Mastery and Enhanced Performance* (Wisdom Publications, Boston, 1991) and *The Fine Arts of Relaxation, Concentration and Meditation* (Wisdom Publications, Boston, 1987) by Dr. Joel and Michelle Levy, founders, Innerwork Technologies, Inc., Seattle, Washington. Reprinted by permission of the authors.

"The Royal Path of Mental Discipline" from *Raja-Yoga* by Swami Vivekananda, edited by Swami Nikhilananda. Copyright © 1955. Published by the Ramakrishna-Vivekananda Center of New York. Reprinted by permission of the publisher.

"Suffering Is Not Enough" from *Being Peace* by Thich Nhat Hanh, Parallax Press, Berkeley, CA 1987. Reprinted by permission of the publisher.

"The Power and Limits of Meditation" from an interview by Catherine Ingram. Reprinted with permission of Ken Wilber.

"Early-Warning Signs for the Detection of Spiritual Blight" originally appeared in the news letter of the Association for Transpersonal Psychology. Reprinted by permission of the author.

"Dancing on the Razor's Edge" by John Welwood. © 1985 by John Welwood.

"Unconditional Love" from *The Power of Unconditional Love* by Ken Keyes, Jr. with P. Keyes. Published by Love Line Books. Reprinted by permission of the author.

About the Editors

Stephan Bodian, M.A., has been editor-in-chief of *Yoga Journal* since 1984. He has practiced yoga and various forms of meditation for nearly twenty-five years, including ten years as a Zen Buddhist monk and teacher. In addition to his work as editor, he has a private practice as a psychotherapist in San Rafael, California, specializing in spiritual and psychological integration. He is also the author of a book of interviews, *Timeless Visions, Healing Voices.*

Georg Feuerstein, Ph.D., is an internationally known yoga scholar who is also a practitioner. He has authored over twenty books, including *Yoga: The Technology of Ecstasy; Sacred Paths; Encyclopedic Dictionary of Yoga; Holy Madness; The Yoga-Sutra of Patanjali; Sacred Sexuality; Wholeness or Transcendence?;* and *The Mystery of Light.* He also is a contributing editor of several national magazines, including *Yoga Journal.*

About Yoga Journal

Yoga Journal is an award-winning bimonthly magazine covering hatha yoga and a range of related topics, including holistic healing and alternative healthcare, transpersonal psychology, new-paradigm thought, bodywork, meditation, and the martial arts, and other approaches to personal and spiritual growth.

At the heart of our work is a vision of a healthy, loving, and harmonious world for all living creatures. To quote our statement of purpose: *"Yoga Journal* is dedicated to communicating, to as broad an audience as possible, the qualities of being that yoga exemplifies: peace, integrity, clarity, and compassion."

To order a one-year (6-issue) subscription to *Yoga Journal*, send your name and complete address, with payment, to:

Yoga Journal
2054 University Avenue, Dept. LY
Berkeley, CA 94704–1082

The cost for a one-year subscription is $18 in the U.S.; $23 in Canada and Mexico; $31 in all other countries.

For Visa/MC orders, send card number and expiration date. All checks or money orders should be in U.S. dollars drawn on a U.S. bank.

Index